T0292035

# The Concise Guide to
# Physiotherapy
## Volume One

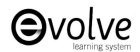

*Commissioning Editor:* Rita Demetriou-Swanwick
*Development Editor:* Catherine Jackson
*Project Manager:* Maggie Johnson
*Designer/Design Direction:* Miles Hitchin
*Illustration Manager:* Tim Ainslie

# The Concise Guide to
# Physiotherapy
## Volume One – Assessment

**Edited by**
*Tim Ainslie MSc GradDipPhys MCSP MMACP*
*Clinical Education Co-ordinator/Senior Lecturer, Physiotherapy Programme,*
*Oxford Brookes University, Oxford, UK*

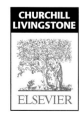

CHURCHILL
LIVINGSTONE

ELSEVIER

Edinburgh  London  New York  Oxford  Philadelphia  St Louis  Sydney  Toronto  2012

# CHURCHILL
# LIVINGSTONE
### ELSEVIER

© 2012 Elsevier Ltd. All rights reserved.

ISBN 978 0 7020 3552 4

ISBN of Vol 2 978 0 7020 4049 8
ISBN of 2-Vol Set 978 0 7020 4048 1

**British Library Cataloguing in Publication Data**
A catalogue record for this book is available from the British Library

**Library of Congress Cataloging in Publication Data**
A catalog record for this book is available from the Library of Congress

**Notices**
Knowledge and best practice in this field are constantly changing. As new research and experience broaden our understanding, changes in research methods, professional practices, or medical treatment may become necessary.

Practitioners and researchers must always rely on their own experience and knowledge in evaluating and using any information, methods, compounds, or experiments described herein. In using such information or methods they should be mindful of their own safety and the safety of others, including parties for whom they have a professional responsibility.

With respect to any drug or pharmaceutical products identified, readers are advised to check the most current information provided (i) on procedures featured or (ii) by the manufacturer of each product to be administered, to verify the recommended dose or formula, the method and duration of administration, and contraindications. It is the responsibility of practitioners, relying on their own experience and knowledge of their patients, to make diagnoses, to determine dosages and the best treatment for each individual patient, and to take all appropriate safety precautions.

To the fullest extent of the law, neither the Publisher nor the authors, contributors, or editors, assume any liability for any injury and/or damage to persons or property as a matter of products liability, negligence or otherwise, or from any use or operation of any methods, products, instructions, or ideas contained in the material herein.

**ELSEVIER** your source for books, journals and multimedia in the health sciences
**www.elsevierhealth.com**

Working together to grow
libraries in developing countries

www.elsevier.com | www.bookaid.org | www.sabre.org

ELSEVIER    BOOK AID International    Sabre Foundation

The publisher's policy is to use paper manufactured from sustainable forests

Printed in China

# Contents

Anne Alexander MSc BSc(Hons) MCSP MMACP
Clinical Specialist Physiotherapist, Hand Therapy and Plastic Surgery Department, John Radcliffe Hospital, Oxford
*Chapter 4 – Burns and plastic surgery*

Rebecca Aston MA MCSP
Specialist Women's Health Physiotherapist, Community PFD Service Team Lead, Homerton Hospital, London
*Chapter 11 – Obstetrics and gynaecology*

Kate Baker BSc(Hons) MCSP
Macmillan Clinical Lead Physiotherapist, Velindre Cancer Centre, Cardiff
*Chapter 12 – Oncology and palliative care*

Sally Braithwaite MCSP
Clinical Professional Clinical Lead, Inclusion Services, Birmingham Community Healthcare NHS Trust, Birmingham
*Chapter 5 – Community paediatrics*

Louise Briggs MSc BSc(Hons) MCSP
AHP Therapy Consultant – Acute Rehabilitation, St George's Health Care NHS Trust, London
*Chapter 7 – Gerontology*

Joanna Camp BSc(Hons) MCSP
Specialist Physiotherapist, National Spinal Injuries Unit, Stoke Mandeville Hospital, Buckinghamshire Healthcare NHS Trust
*Chapter 16 – Spinal cord injuries*

Maureen Carter BA MCSP
Retired Senior Physiotherapist in Community and Intermediate Care, Croydon, Surrey
*Chapter 6 – Community physiotherapy*

Mark L. Clemence MPhil GradDipPhys MCSP
Clinical Specialist Physiotherapist, South Devon Healthcare NHS Trust, Devon
*Chapter 15 – Rheumatology*

Mary Jane Cole MSc GradDipPhys MCSP ACE
Senior Lecturer, Practice Education, Kingston University and St George's University of London, London
*Chapter 2 – Amputee rehabilitation*

Karen Edwards MSc MCSP
Clinical Specialist Physiotherapist Great Ormond Street Hospital, London
*Chapter 5 – Community paediatrics*

Susie Grady MSc BSc(Hons) MCSP
Aquatic Therapy Team Leader, The Gardens and Jacob Centres, Hertfordshire
*Chapter 3 – Aquatic physiotherapy*

Caroline Griffiths GradDipPhys MCSP
Professional Lead, Physiotherapy, Oxford Health NHS Foundation Trust, Oxford
*Chapter 10 – Mental health*

Vicki Harding PhD MCSP
Research and Clinical Specialist Physiotherapist, INPUT Pain Management Programme, St Thomas' Hospital, London
*Chapter 13 – Pain management*

Nicola Harmer GradDipPhys MCSP
Highly Specialist Physiotherapist/Directorate Manual Handling Advisor, Directorate of Learning Disability Services, Abertawe Bro Morgannwg University Health Board
*Chapter 8 – Learning disabilities*

Scott Hawthorne BAppSc MCSP MAPA
Band 7 Physiotherapist, Acute Spinal Injuries Physiotherapy Lead, National Spinal Injuries Centre, Stoke Mandeville Hospital, Buckinghamshire Healthcare NHS Trust
*Chapter 16 – Spinal cord injuries*

Andrea Hounsell MSc BSc(Hons) MCSP
Physiotherapy Team Leader, Directorate of Learning Disability Services, Abertawe Bro Morgannwg University Health Board
*Chapter 8 – Learning disabilities*

Anne Jackson PhD MSc BA(Hons) MCSP
English Networks Programme Manager, Chartered Society of Physiotherapy, London
*Chapter 3 – Aquatic physiotherapy*

Deborah Jackson MSc BSc(Hons) MCSP
Clinical Specialist Physiotherapist, Great Ormond Street Hospital, London
*Chapter 1 – Acute paediatrics*

Captain Mark Jenkins MSc BSc(Hons) MCSP RAMC
Officer in Command, Primary Care Rehabilitation Facility, Wellington Barracks, London
*Chapter 14 – Rehabilitation*

Lesley Katchburian MSc MCSP
Clinical Specialist Physiotherapist (Neurodisability), The Wolfson Neurodisability Service, Great Ormond Street Hospital, London
*Chapter 1 – Acute paediatrics*

**Karen Livingstone MCSP GradDipPhys**
Clinical Specialist Physiotherapist in Oncology and Palliative Care, St Ann's Hospice, Neil Cliffe Centre, Wythenshawe Hospital, Manchester
*Chapter 12 – Oncology and palliative care*

**Marion Main MA MCSP**
Dubowitz Neuromuscular Centre, Great Ormond Street Hospital, London
*Chapter 1 – Acute paediatrics*

**Mike Maynard GradDipPhys HT**
Clinical Lead in Aquatic Physiotherapy, United Lincolnshire Hospitals
*Chapter 3 – Aquatic physiotherapy*

**Aileen McCartney MSc BSc(Hons) MCSP**
Senior Physiotherapist, Specialist Palliative Care, Wisdom Hospital, Rochester, Kent
*Chapter 12 – Oncology and palliative care*

**Doreen McClurg PhD MCSP**
Reader, NMAHP Research Unit, Glasgow Caledonian University, Glasgow
*Chapter 11 – Obstetrics and gynaecology*

**John McLennan PG Cert Pain Management GradDipPhys MCSP**
Lead Physiotherapist, Lothian Chronic Pain Service, Edinburgh
*Chapter 13 – Pain management*

**Clare Nickols MSc BSc(Hons) MCSP**
In-Patient Team Leader/Deputy Physiotherapy Manager, Heatherwood Hospital, Ascot, Berkshire
*Chapter 9 – Medicine*

**Jayne Nixon BSc(Hons) Dip Sport Ex Med MCSP**
Clinical Specialist and Clinical Lead – Lower Limbs Team, Defence Medical Rehabilitation Centre, Headley Court, Epsom, Surrey
*Chapter 14 – Rehabilitation*

**Siobhan O'Mahony PGDip Health Services Management GradDipPhys MCSP**
Physiotherapy Manager, St Patrick's Hospital (Cork) Ltd, Cork, Ireland
*Chapter 12 – Oncology and palliative care*

**Ankie Postma GradDipPhys**
Basildon Hospital, Essex
*Chapter 3    Aquatic physiotherapy*

**Davina Richardson MSc BSc(Hons) MCSP**
Clinical Lead Therapist, Neurosciences, Imperial College Healthcare NHS Trust, London
*Chapter 14 – Rehabilitation*

**Karen A.J. Rix GradDipPhys MCSP**
Clinical Team Leader, Community Intermediate Care Service, London
*Chapter 6 – Community physiotherapy*

**Andrew Rolls MSC BSC(Hons) MCSP**
Head of Sports Medicine, West Ham United Football Club, London
*Chapter 14 – Rehabilitation*

**Janine Rutland GradDipPhys MCSP**
Community Paediatric Physiotherapist, The Avenue School, Reading, Berkshire
*Chapter 5 – Community paediatrics*

**Josie Scerri BSc(Hons) MCSP**
Senior Physiotherapist, Neurodisability Service, Great Ormond Street Hospital, London
*Chapter 1 – Acute paediatrics*

**Warren Sheehan BPhty MCSP**
Senior physiotherapist, John Radcliffe Hospital, Oxford
*Chapter 17 – Trauma orthopaedics*

**Sara Smith GradDipPhys PGCert(ClinEd) MCSP**
Amputee Therapy Team Leader, Rehabilitation Gym, Douglas Bader Centre, Queen Mary's Hospital, London
*Chapter 2 – Amputee rehabilitation*

**Sue Standing MSc MCSP**
Lead Physiotherapist, Hampshire Partnership Foundation Trust, Southampton
*Chapter 8 – Learning disabilities*

**Robyn Stiger MSc BSc(Hons) MCSP**
Associate Lecturer, Physiotherapy Undergraduate Programme, Oxford Brookes University, Oxford
*Chapter 1 – Acute paediatrics*

**Catherine Stringer BSc(Hons) BEd MCSP**
Senior Musculoskeletal Physiotherapist/
Hydrotherapy, Physiotherapy Department,
Good Hope Hospital, West Midlands
*Chapter 3 – Aquatic physiotherapy*

**Clara Upson BSc(Hons) MCSP**
Advanced Physiotherapist Burns and Plastic
Surgery Stoke Mandeville Hospital,
Buckinghamshire Healthcare NHS Trust
*Chapter 4 – Burns and plastic surgery*

**Anna Vines BSc(Hons) MCSP**
Senior Physiotherapist, John Radcliffe
Hospital, Oxford
*Chapter 17 – Trauma orthopaedics*

**Yvonne Wren GradDipPhys**
Retired Clinical Therapy Lead for Intermediate
Care, Southwark; Retired Specialist Lecturer,
University of East London, London
*Chapter 6 – Community physiotherapy*

Contributors

# Preface

Students and graduate physiotherapists report feeling underprepared when entering an unfamiliar practice area for the first time. The core areas of musculoskeletal, neurology and cardio-respiratory tend to be covered in depth in the university as students are prepared for practice placements and it is often the 'non-core' areas such as burns and plastic surgery or palliative care that can cause a student to feel anxious and underprepared. Written by specialists from the 'non-core' areas of practice the two volumes of this book aim to provide the student or graduate with an insight into the philosophy of approach that needs to be taken in either the assessment (volume 1) or the treatment (volume 2) of the individual in these placement areas. The material provides an entry level of knowledge with the expectation that the reader will access more 'in-depth' information, in order to supplement the material provided in the two volumes and on-line resources.

Tim Ainslie

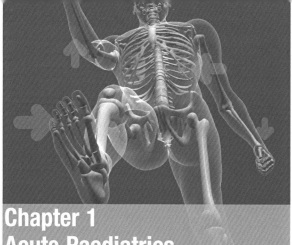

# Chapter 1
# Acute Paediatrics
## Neuromuscular disorders

## Clinical features

Paediatric neuromuscular (NM) disorders are a diverse group of progressive conditions, characterised by muscle weakness and contractures that include the neck, spine, and jaw.

- Other features of NM disorders:
- spinal deformity, e.g. scoliosis or increased lumbar lordosis
- neck and spine rigidity
- varying degrees of functional limitation
- abnormal gait patterns and/or associated foot postures
- toe walking
- foot drop
- frequent falls
- pes cavus
- developmental delay
- lack of independent mobility
- fatigue
- respiratory involvement
- cardiac problems
- calf hypertrophy, e.g. Duchenne muscular dystrophy (DMD)
- muscle wasting, e.g. type III spinal muscular atrophy (SMA)
- facial weakness
- winging scapulae
- cramp or pain, particularly on exercise.

Children with neuromuscular disorders do not have increased tone, apart from a few who have very rare disorders, or increased tone due to a non-related condition: e.g. an unrelated hemiplegia.

Hypotonic as a term should be avoided, as the terms weak and low tone are frequently used interchangeably; they are not the same.

The conditions vary in many ways, but often the greatest concern for therapists is the rate of progression of symptoms.

An important consideration is the effect of growth; while the underlying condition may be slowly progressive, the increase in height and weight can have a major effect on motor performance and function.

It is important to understand that progressive neuromuscular disorders are frightening for parents and children. The children, especially the weakest ones, will be wary of strangers and may need time before they will co-operate with assessment.

## Assessment

This will vary according to age, function, whether an infant, child or teenager is being assessed for the first time or if they are being reviewed.

### Subjective assessment

- During the initial assessment, an overview of the onset, progression and major functional difficulties needs to be established.
- Is there any family history of muscle disorders or developmental delay?
- Are the problems getting worse, improving or staying the same?
- If function or power has deteriorated, has this happened gradually or rapidly?
- Is the child experiencing symptoms of nocturnal hypoventilation?
- Weaker children with neuromuscular conditions often suffer from nocturnal hypoventilation, i.e. they under-breathe when asleep.
- To ascertain whether a child may be developing this problem, the following questions should be asked:
- Do they sleep badly (some complain of nightmares)?
- Do they have morning headaches?
- Do they find it difficult to wake or are slow to wake?
- Do they demonstrate morning anorexia (refuse to eat breakfast)?
- Do they experience daytime sleepiness or lack of concentration at school?

### Babies and infants

- The following need to be considered when assessing babies or infants:
- Duration of pregnancy; full term?
- Did the baby move appropriately in utero?
- Did they require any respiratory or feeding support in the neonatal period?
- Is the baby making progress in their development?
- Do they have good head control and have they reached their appropriate motor milestones?
- Does the baby interact with parents and their environment?
- Does the baby have good general health or are they prone to chest infections?
- Was the baby born with or have they developed any contractures?

## Ambulant children

- When assessing an ambulant child the following need to be considered:
- What age did they walk independently?
- If walking is deteriorating, when did this begin?
- Is walking slower than expected?
- How far can the child walk in terms of time or distance? It may be necessary to specify on a 'good day', or when allowed to go at their own pace.
- What limits walking; falls, fatigue, pain?
- What are the major functional difficulties? for example; climbing stairs, getting up from the floor and running.
- Outdoors, can they manage kerbs and slopes?
- Does the child get cramp or pain: and if so where? Are there precipitating factors? Is it most apparent after exercise?
- Have they had previous factures or surgery?
- Are they using any splints or orthotics?
- What exercise and activity do they do?
- Do they swim, ride a bicycle, play football, dance, do gymnastics or participate in any other activities?
- Do they play any musical instruments?
- Do they join in during PE sessions at school?

## Non-ambulant children

- When assessing non-ambulant children the following need to be considered:
- Can they sit independently?
- Did they ever walk and if so, when did they lose the ability?
- How do they mobilise?
- Have they any specialist equipment?
- How much are parents carrying or lifting them?
- What are the access issues at home or outside at school or nursery?

## Considerations for teenagers

- Onset of disorders in the teenage years can be especially hard – being a teenager is difficult enough!
- There may be conflicting history with parents or playing down of symptoms to feign normality.

## Objective assessment

Assessment of infants, children and adolescents will focus on the evaluation of muscle power, joint range and contractures, mobility, posture and function.

In some centres, respiratory function is tested by physiotherapists.

For babies and infants, an assessment of developmental milestones is needed.

## Development

- Does the baby have good head control?
- Are they trying to roll?
- Can they get into sitting, or safely lie down once placed in sitting?
- Do they get distressed when placed prone?

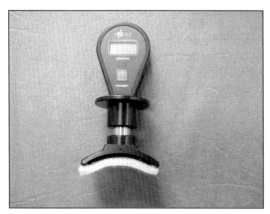

**Figure 1.1 Hand-held dynamometer.** *With kind permission of Citec, www.citec.nu.*

- Do they/did they crawl and/or bottom shuffle?
- Can they take weight through their legs when placed in standing?

## Muscle power:

- Assessment of muscle power in clinical practice on the whole follows the MRC grading/Oxford scale of 0–5 (MRC 1976).
- Standardised starting positions must be used to ensure reproducibility.
- Pure movements are tested at the neck, trunk, hips, knees and ankles, shoulders, elbows forearms and wrists.
- Rotation movements are not tested, as they are not pure movements. Although strong and often used to compensate for weakness, it is difficult to separate the components of the movement.
- Objective measurement of force using a hand-held dynamometer, also known as myometry, has been shown to be more reliable as a means of measuring muscle power in children (Wadsworth et al 1987) (Figure 1.1).

## Joint contractures

- Contractures may be present which can influence joint range of motion.
- Caused by shortening of the muscle and other structures around the joint.
- The muscles can be:
- Fibrosed, due to underlying disease
- Shortened, through lack of movement or muscle imbalance
- Shortened, due to repeated poor posture or a reduced repertoire of movement.
- There are children who have joint hypermobility or a combination of hypermobility and contractures.
- Marked hypermobility can be as debilitating as contractures and should be recorded.
- Contractures are more severe and widespread in non-ambulant children.

- They are apparent at birth in many of the congenital muscular dystrophies, but can occur in all of the neuromuscular disorders over time.
- The site of contractures can be related to the underlying pattern of muscle weakness and to the functional level of the child (ambulant or non-ambulant).
- Contractures are important where they interfere with function.
- The most frequently encountered contractures are:
- Hip flexion
- Ankle, loss of dorsiflexion
- Iliotibial band (ITB)
- Elbow
- Long finger flexors
- Loss of supination
- Knee
- Neck and spinal rigidity
- Mid-foot, leading to pes cavus deformity.

## Measurement of joint range

- Commonly joint range is measured using goniometry.
- Standardised starting positions and measuring methods need to be defined to ensure repeatability.
- It is also very important to know what constitutes 'normal' range when considering the presence of reduced joint range.
- Neck range of movement and spinal mobility are routinely assessed.
- Hamstring range is measured routinely recording the popliteal angle. However tighter hamstrings are a prerequisite for children with pelvic weakness, to ensure the highest level of function.
- Hamstring tightness is not considered to be a problem unless it is associated with collagen disorders, e.g. Ullrich congenital muscular dystrophy (CMD) or Bethlem CMD.

## Mobility

- When a child is ambulant, timed tests are used to provide quantitative measures of mobility.
- With the timed 10 metres, the child is instructed to 'go' as fast as they can.
- More recently, the 6 minute walk test (6MWT) has been introduced (Li et al 2005). Distance is measured over a course, recommended to be 25 metres long, and continued for 6 minutes with the distance walked being recorded.

## Posture

- Descriptions of neck/spine posture in sitting and neck/spine and leg posture in standing are recorded.
- X-rays are taken when necessary.
- The following need to be noted in sitting and standing:
- In sitting, is there a scoliosis, kyphosis, increased lordosis in the spine?
- Is there spinal rotation or rib humps?
- Are the shoulders level?
- Is there winging of the scapulae?

- Is the pelvis level?
- Are waist creases and contours symmetrical?
- Is the head held straight or tilted?
- In standing, is the pelvis level, and does the spinal posture change.
- Is there asymmetry of the legs?
- Does the child have normal foot posture or pes cavus/pes planus?

## Function

- Function in neuromuscular disorders is assessed using a functional scale.
- The scales used will depend on the preferences of the centre, the diagnosis and the functional level of the child.
- The main areas that are tested:
- lifting the head
- rolling
- getting to sitting from lying
- crawling
- standing up from the floor
- standing on one leg
- hopping
- jumping
- getting up and down steps/stairs.

### Teenagers

- For a teenager reviewed over many years, who has never walked or lost ambulation, assessing power and contractures will provide information that they and their parents/carers will already know, i.e. that they are weaker and more contracted.

### Parents and siblings

- It is important to consider whether this is a disorder that may also affect a parent or sibling.
- The following signs may be observed in parents and siblings and may help to give clues to help the formation of a diagnosis:
- Elbow contractures, TA tightness, long finger flexor tightness (Bethlem CMD)
- Facial weakness (fascioscapular-humeral MD)
- Calf hypertrophy (carrier of DMD – females)
- Pes cavus (Charcot–Marie–Tooth).

## Summary

- Weakness and contractures are the major barriers to function.
- Many children will have or develop respiratory compromise.
- Many children will have spinal asymmetry that may require corrective surgery.
- It is not appropriate to keep assessing power and contractures in the older, weakest non-ambulant teenagers.
- Progressive disorders are frightening and the fears and anxieties of the parents and children will need to be managed in a sympathetic manner.

# Musculoskeletal

- Assessment of a child requires an understanding of normal growth and development of the musculoskeletal system as well as an awareness of potential red flags.
- It is important to involve the whole team, family/carers and the child in all discussions from the outset, so that consequent management aims are realistic, relevant and achievable.
- Whilst both adults and children will attend the initial assessment with an element of anxiety, this tends to predominate in children and it can be harder to reason with them.
- Ensure that the environment and assessment are as non-threatening and friendly as possible.
- Assessment should be undertaken with the parent/carer in close proximity, often with the child on their lap.
- Clear explanations should be given before undertaking any testing procedures.

## Subjective assessment

### Birth history

- Health of mother and baby during pregnancy including any medication taken
- Gestational age of baby
- Labour and delivery process
- Postnatal problems or care needed.

### Development

- Unusual childhood illnesses
- Developmental milestones: e.g. at what age did the infant first roll, sit or walk (Sheridan et al 2008)
- Information regarding school (as appropriate):

### Family history

- Number, age and health of siblings
- Similar presentations within family.

### Parent/carer concerns

- Take their concerns seriously, as their instincts are often accurate and may help focus your assessment.

### Pain

- The manner in which a child expresses pain will depend on their age and may manifest in the following ways:
- Altered sleep patterns and feeding
- Distress on handling or movement of the affected area
- Continuous crying in the presence of severe pain
- Avoidance of moving the affected part or altered function, e.g. limping
- A child may only be able to give a vague description and localisation of pain

- Be aware of underplaying or exaggeration of symptoms in adolescents wanting to either participate in or avoid sports or other activities.
- Various pain assessment tools are available depending on the age and cognitive ability of the child, e.g. pain faces scale (Hicks et al 2001), paediatric pain profile (UCL, ICH, RCNI 2003).

## Objective assessment

### Baby

- The most rapid period of growth and development occurs in the first 18 months of life.
- By 2 years a child is already approximately half their adult height.
- A fastidious approach is vital as infants tend to be unable to indicate where problems are or to comply with assessment.
- Undress the whole child, irrespective of the referral, to avoid missing any orthopaedic problems or diagnostic clues.

#### Observation

- Overall size and proportion of child
- Count number, and check separation, of toes (indications of congenital abnormalities)
- Asymmetries (postural deformities are frequent in neonates and may occur as a result of intrauterine pressure or positioning)
- Any baby with asymmetries may have an increased risk of hip dysplasia
- In particular, note any:
- Plagiocephaly (flattening of the skull)
- Torticollis (asymmetry of neck movement)
- Postural foot deformities

#### Movement and functional strength

- Spontaneous movement patterns
- Reduced movement of any joint can be indicative of septic arthritis
- Reduced movement of an upper limb may indicate Erb's palsy
- Passive range of movement
- Joint range will change with age and so the therapist should refer to texts for normal ranges in infants
- In the newborn, joint position will be affected by intrauterine position, i.e. lateral hip rotation, knee and hip flexion contractures, and excessive dorsiflexion are common (Staheli 2008).

#### Spine check

- A baby's spine should be straight with a single C-shaped curve. Scoliosis is always abnormal in a baby and should be investigated.
- Look for skin changes such as hairy patches, birth marks, café-au-lait patches and skin dimples over the spine indicating underlying spinal problems, e.g. spina bifida occulta, spinal dysraphism or neurofibromatosis.

### Hip screening

- Babies in the UK are routinely screened for hip dysplasia; however developmental dysplasia of the hip (DDH) is occasionally missed.
- Hips should be checked for:
- Range of abduction
- Asymmetric skin folds
- Apparent femoral shortening
- Ortolani and Barlow tests for instability (Barlow 1962; Ortolani 1976; AAP 2000).

## Child (age 2½ until adolescence)

- During this time growth and development continue, but at a slower rate than in infancy. However, because childhood lasts so long, the majority of growth and development occurs during this period.

### Range of movement

- Active and passive joint ROM:
- Note joint laxity, defined by examining range of extension of ankles, knees, elbows, wrist, thumbs and fingers
- Excessive laxity is a contributor to the pathogenesis of hip dysplasia, genu valgum, recurrent patella dislocation and pes planus. It can also provide an alert to other problems, e.g. Ehlers–Danlos or Marfan's syndrome and osteogenesis imperfecta.
- Muscle length (popliteal angle, Silfverskiöld test).
- Bony rotational profiles:
- Tibial torsion
- Thigh foot angle
- Femoral anteversion.

### Muscle power

- Medical Research Council Scale (MRC 1976) or Hammersmith functional motor scale, as appropriate (Main et al 2003).

### Limb lengths (and girth)

- Tape measure:
- In the presence of congenital deformities, functional leg length discrepancy measurement is taken from the ASIS to the base of the heel.
- Galeazzi sign:
- Child supine, hips and knees flexed with feet aligned, assess whether leg length difference is from femur or tibia.
- Blocks:
- It is often more accurate to ask the child to place their shortened limb on blocks of differing heights until the pelvis is aligned or the child feels level.

### Joint stability

- Abnormal joint shape and absence of ligaments are frequent features of congenital deformities.

Gait

- Normal gait does not mature until around the 7th year.
- Check shoes for contact areas and wear patterns.
- Video, Physician rating scale, Edinburgh gait scale (Maathuis et al 2005).
- Gait laboratory may be helpful for children with neuromuscular disorders, preoperative planning and assessing postoperative outcomes.

Normal variants

- Children vary in shape, size and rate of development and therefore ranges of normal are not easily defined.
- Many children referred to orthopaedic clinics have nothing wrong with them and most variations are outgrown (Bennett 2002).
- An aim of the assessment in these children is therefore to exclude abnormality, e.g. using 5S's (Jones and Hill 2000):
  - *Symmetry*
  a If both limbs are affected equally, the presentation is more likely to be normal physiology and management is to monitor.
  b Severe or asymmetric deformity warrants referral for further investigation.
  - *Symptoms*
  a If the child is not complaining of any symptoms or experiencing functional difficulties, intervention is unlikely to be needed.
  - *Stiffness*
  a Joint stiffness in a growing child requires further investigation.
  - *Systemic disease*
  a Inflammatory and metabolic conditions can affect skeletal growth, therefore establish whether a child is medically well.
  - *Skeletal dysplasia*
  a Growth charts determine whether height and weight are within normal proportions. Unusual facial features may also indicate a dysplasia.
  b Deformity in children will never be truly static due to ongoing growth, therefore careful and regular monitoring is required.

## Motor disorders

- Motor disorders can be due to:
- Cerebral palsy (Box 1.1)
- Genetic disorders, e.g. hereditary spastic paraplegia
- Metabolic disorders, e.g. mitochondrial disorders, leucodystrophies
- Acquired brain injury.
- In order to share a common language and aid communication about a child's difficulties, the child should be provided with a diagnosis whenever possible and given a classification which describes their motor function:
- Distribution: Unilateral, bilateral or total body involvement
- Type: Spastic, hypotonic, dyskinetic (dystonic or athetoid) or ataxic
- Severity: If the child has cerebral palsy, there are specific tools available to determine severity levels (Box 1.2).

---

**Box 1.1** Definition of cerebral palsy

**Cerebral palsy**

- The term used for a group of non-progressive disorders of movement and posture caused by abnormal development or damage to the motor control centres of the brain
- The most prevalent cause for motor disorders in childhood with 2–3 per 1000 live births (Heinen et al 2009)
- CP is caused by events before, during or after birth (up to 2 years of age)
- The abnormalities of muscle control that define CP are often accompanied by other neurological and physical abnormalities
- The non-motor features that accompany the muscle control issues of CP include:
- Sensory disturbance (vision, hearing and touch)
- Feeding difficulties
- Dysarthria
- Drooling
- Bladder dysfunction
- Epilepsy
- Hydrocephalus
- Learning difficulties
- Behavioural problems

---

**Box 1.2** Descriptors of severity in cerebral palsy

- The Gross Motor Function Classification System (GMFCS), defines five levels of motor ability (www.canchild.com)
- The Manual Ability Classification System (MACS) defines five levels of hand function (www.macs.nu)
- The Functional Mobility Scale (FMS) assesses mobility in children across 3 distances (www.rch.org.au/gait)

---

## Assessment

- Children are usually referred for a secondary/tertiary neurological opinion within a hospital setting, generally for consideration of the diagnosis and prognosis.
- The physiotherapist in this setting works as a member of a multidisciplinary team, which may consist of a paediatric neurologist and/or neurodisability paediatrician.
- The WHO International Classification of Functioning, Disability and Health (http://www.who.int/classifications/icf/icfapptraining/en/index.html) is a framework for measuring health and disability and should be adhered to or considered when carrying out an assessment (Appendix 1.1).

### Subjective

- Before starting the assessment, it is useful to understand the questions, concerns and priorities of the family.

## Birth history

- Acquire as much information as possible from the referrer to reduce the duplication of assessment questions and distress this can cause repeating what is often a traumatic neonatal history.

- Prenatal and perinatal history should be obtained if it is not available, including an account of pregnancy and birth history to ensure that the presentation of the child fits with the possible causes of brain injury, e.g. preterm presentation or hypoxic injury at term.

## Investigations

- Early ultrasound, CT or MRI scans provide information about the child's brain development in the early neonatal phase and later childhood.

- Blood tests including genetic testing can exclude metabolic or hereditary causes.

- A baseline hip X-ray particularly with the more severely affected children (GMFCS III–V) should be performed, especially when there is a description of pain or asymmetry.

- Children at risk of hip subluxation require regular pelvic X-rays and date of last imaging should be known.

## Past medical history

- Additional problems may influence a child's tone, e.g.:
- Previous surgery
- Ventriculoperitoneal shunt in situ following treatment for hydrocephalus
- Associated problems, e.g. seizures
- Feeding problems, reflux, percutaneous endoscopic gastrostomy (PEG) feeding following gastrostomy or swallowing issues
- Frequent chest infections?
- Difficulty managing saliva?
- Constipation?

## Communication

- How does the child communicate?
- Visual impairments?
- Hearing issues?
- Recent hearing check?

## Drug history/medication

- Current medication
- Previous trials of medication and their outcome, e.g. child with spasticity and effects of Baclofen?

## Family history

- Similar problems in the immediate and extended family?
- Are the parents consanguineous?

## Motor milestones

- A detailed developmental history is required considering developmental milestones appropriate for the child's age (Sheridan et al 2008).

- It is also important to look out for any episodes of deterioration or regression.
- A progressive neuromuscular disorder is not usually associated with CP; however, a deterioration in mobility may be noticed around puberty.

## Current functional ability

- Usual mobility at home, in school and generally?
- Do they use aids?
- Assistance required when walking?
- Daily routine in and out of school, e.g. participation in PE, after-school activities?
- ADLs, e.g. feeding, dressing, will give an indication of fine motor skills.
- Favourite activities? This enables understanding of the child and their cognitive ability.
- Is there a statement of special educational needs outlining how many hours of support they have?
- Consider the child as a whole person functioning within a family or school environment.

## Professionals involved

- Which professionals are currently involved and to what degree?
- Previous interventions, e.g. botulinum toxin injections for spasticity.

## Orthotics and equipment

- Current orthotics and equipment?
- Previously tried, e.g. sleep system?
- Current 24-hour postural management programme.

## Objective assessment

- Children are often apprehensive in a hospital setting, take time to observe the child whilst sitting with their parent or carer.
- It is also possible to assess much of a child's functional ability whilst they play.
- It may be possible to video the assessment or components such as gait (written consent must be obtained).

## Observation

- This should be done with the child in lying, sitting and standing (Box 1.3)

## Functional ability

- Assessment of younger children may focus on floor mobility, whereas higher-functioning older children may need the focus to be on gait or higher functions, e.g. running.

## Standardised functional tests

- For extensive assessment of gross motor skills, the gross motor function measure (GMFM) GMFM-88 or GMFM-66 can be used.
- Upper limb standardised functional assessment of bimanual function can be evaluated using the Assisting Hand Assessment (Krumlinde-Sundholm et al 2007), SHUEE, Physicians Rating Scale (Davids et al 2006).

---

**Box 1.3** Observation of the child

**Lying**

- Posture
- Check for asymmetry, dystonic posturing, increased tone and use of base of support
- Abilities
- Check if moving limbs, head and trunk against gravity; assess gross motor skills and transitions, e.g. forearm support in prone, rolling
- Observe
- what they can do, how they perform the activity, what is limiting them from achieving the next motor milestone

**Sitting**

- Postural influences
- e.g. tight hamstrings may cause posterior tilt of the pelvis; dystonic spasms; athetoid movements; independent sitting
- Observe
- balance reactions, saving reactions, sitting on the edge of a plinth (with feet supported and unsupported), mat sitting looking at the ability to weight shift and reach laterally out of the base of support
- Check the spine
- while sitting on the edge of a plinth, provide gentle traction through the spine to see whether low trunk tone is contributing to a postural scoliosis, forward slump test can also help differentiate between structural or postural curve. Request a spinal X-ray if in doubt, especially if pelvic and hip mobility is limited.

**Standing**

- Posture
- shoulder and pelvic levels, foot posture and how correctable this is
- Static and dynamic balance. While observing single leg stance, check balance reactions around ankle if any, if not, where compensation occurs
- Pelvic control
- Ability to jump and hop, any associated reactions or dystonic posturing?

---

## Muscle power

- Formal testing may be difficult when a child is very young or if cognition is affected.
- In these cases look at functional activities, e.g. rising from sitting to standing or repeated toe standing.
- If the child is able to you can examine their ability to activate and sustain muscle contraction using the 5 point MRC scale (MRC 1981).

## Selective muscle control

- Selective muscle control will influence the gait cycle and the child's general mobility.
- If a child has poor selective control, they will use 'mass patterns' to move, e.g. hip flexion with knee flexion and dorsiflexion, followed by hip and knee extension with plantarflexion.

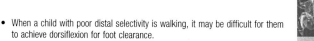

- When a child with poor distal selectivity is walking, it may be difficult for them to achieve dorsiflexion for foot clearance.
- There are various standardised assessment tools to assess selective muscle control:
- SCALE (Fowler et al 2009)
- Selective motor control grading scale description (Gage et al, 2009)
- SMC (Selective Motor Control) (Boyd and Graham 1999).

## Measuring joint range of movement (ROM), bony torsion, muscle length and muscle tone

- Measurement of ROM includes joint range and muscle length, bony torsion and tone across a muscle using a modified Tardieu assessment (Gracies et al 2010).
- Goniometry should be used, adopting standardised measuring positions.

### Muscle tone

- It is important to differentiate between spasticity, rigidity and dystonia, as well as describing the severity of the abnormal tone.
- The hypertonia assessment tool can be used to help differentiate (Appendix 1.2).
- The Ashworth/Modified Ashworth (Bohannon and Smith 1986) and Tardieu/ modified Tardieu scales are tools that the physiotherapist can use to measure spasticity/rigidity, dynamic spasticity and the 'catch'.
- Deep tendon reflexes are indicators of altered tone.
- Dystonia is usually seen at rest, spasticity increases during activity.
- Dystonic limbs return to a fixed posture and are mostly observed in hands and feet.
- Clinically dystonic postures are usually described but dystonia scales do exist such as the Barry Albright Dystonia Scale (Barry et al 1999) and the Burke–Fahn–Marsden Scale.
- Formal dystonia scales may be useful clinically if assessing the effects of therapeutic or medical/surgical intervention.

### Gait

- Video recording of gait enables the therapist to observe gait without a child having to repeat an activity.
- Video enables comparison of gait pre- and post-intervention.
- Children should be ideally dressed in tight-fitting shorts and if possible a tight-fitting vest to observe the trunk and pelvis.
- Observe general stability, e.g. walking with or without a walking aid, orthoses or shoes.
- How well does the child manoeuvre and stop and start.
- Scales designed to be used with video analysis include the observational gait scale (Mackey et al 2003) and the Edinburgh visual gait score (Read et al 2003).

## Cardiorespiratory

- Respiratory infections are a leading cause of illness in children and are one of the main reasons that a child might be admitted to hospital.

**Table 1.1** Paediatric age ranges

| | |
|---|---|
| Neonate | A baby less than 44 weeks of age from date of conception |
| Infant | Up to 12 months of age |
| Child | 30 months–12 years of age |
| Adolescent | 13–16 years of age |

**Table 1.2** Common causes of acute respiratory failure in children

| Neonate | Children under 2 years | Children over 2 years |
|---|---|---|
| Prematurity | Bronchopneumonia | Asthma |
| Respiratory distress syndrome (RDS) | Respiratory syncytial virus (RSV) bronchiolitis | CNS infection, e.g. meningitis |
| Asphyxia (lack of oxygen before, during or after birth) | Asthma | Trauma |
| Aspiration pneumonia, e.g. meconium aspiration | Laryngotracheobronchitis (croup) | |
| | Foreign body aspiration, e.g. food, wrapper, toy | |
| | Congenital heart or lung abnormalities | |

- There are many anatomical and physiological differences when comparing the respiratory system of infants and children to adults.
- Children are more vulnerable to respiratory infections and complications than adults.
- The undergraduate student or recently qualified physiotherapist working in paediatrics will require support from an experienced paediatric physiotherapist in order to develop the necessary skills and techniques required to assess and manage infants and children.
- Paediatrics covers a wide age range (Table 1.1).
- Common reasons why an infant or child might develop respiratory failure, become acutely unwell and require admission to a neonatal, general paediatric or specialist cardiac intensive care unit can also be categorised by age (Table 1.2).

## Assessment of the infant and child

- Assessment needs to be concise, to ensure that there is minimal disruption to the infant or child, but also effective.
- Much of the assessment can be performed prior to disturbing the child.
- The 'hands on' part of the objective assessment and treatment can be grouped together.
- This is particularly useful when assessing acutely ill children in intensive care.

- Before assessing, an explanation of why physiotherapy is required and what it will entail should be given and consent obtained from parents or carers.
- It is equally important to engage the child depending on their age and level of consciousness.
- Although parents are able to refuse physiotherapy, they seldom do in practice.
- Ideally the child should be rested and in as normal a state as possible to be able to tolerate physiotherapy.
- If the child is crying because of hunger, pain, or a full nappy, it is likely to exacerbate respiratory symptoms and the child is unlikely to tolerate treatment.
- To avoid the baby being sick and possibly aspirating, treatment should be commenced just before a feed, if possible, allowing sufficient time for its completion prior to that feed.
- This is important as optimal nutrition is critical in sick babies.

## Subjective assessment

- Have you treated this patient before?
- If not, are they new to the service or have they been treated by someone else on the team?
- Medical notes are often extensive and bulky, important information may be missed, therefore it is important to communicate with the people involved with the child, e.g. members of the medical team, nursing team and parents or carers.
- If the child has a history of chronic respiratory disease they may have physiotherapy at home, therefore it will be necessary to communicate with the community physiotherapy team.
- Information from the medical notes/ward round/medical discussion:
- Why has the child been admitted to hospital/PICU/NICU?
- Is this their first admission?
- Do they have a history of respiratory disease or are they usually fit and well?
- How long has the child been in hospital/PICU/NICU?
- Is the child's condition improving, deteriorating or stable?
- Have there been any relevant changes overnight or within the last few hours affecting the stability of the child's condition?
- What investigations have been reported on or are due to be undertaken. Does this affect physiotherapy treatment options?
- What is the patient's medical plan for the day (e.g. extubation, CT scan etc.)?
- Information from nurse in charge of the patient:
- How well is the child tolerating handling and interventions?
- If they require suction, what type of suction is needed and when were they last suctioned?
- What is coming up on suction and how frequently does it need to be performed?
- When was the child last repositioned? What was the reason for doing this?
- What is the nursing plan for the day?
- Previous physiotherapy intervention.
- This information may be obtained from the medical notes or from discussion with physiotherapy colleagues.

- Critically ill children may require additional out-of-hours physiotherapy intervention.
- To act in the best interests of a child, it is important to establish:
- What main problems were identified by previous physiotherapy assessment?
- What treatment techniques were used and why?
- Did the patient tolerate these techniques and were they effective?
- What did the physiotherapist suggest post treatment and was that plan carried out?
- Information from the child's parents/carers:
- What is the child normally able to achieve from a developmental point of view? Remember to put this in context with what would be appropriate for their age.
- Do they have physiotherapy at home?
- If yes, why do they need it, how frequently is it performed and by whom?
- If the child has a chronic respiratory illness (excess secretions) or a neuromuscular disease affecting their respiratory muscles (poor cough strength), they might require daily physiotherapy which has been taught to the parents by the community team.
- They may also use physiotherapy adjuncts like a PEP mask, flutter or cough assist machine.

## Objective assessment (prior to disturbing the patient)

- Consider what equipment and monitoring systems are being used?
- Is the child breathing spontaneously, using some kind of breathing support, e.g. CPAP, or are they intubated and mechanically ventilated?
- How awake are they?
- Are they on any sedation or pharmacologically paralysing drugs?
- What drains and lines are in situ? Identify where they are and why they are there, e.g. a chest drain for a pneumothorax.
- Look for cardiovascular system trends on the observations chart:
- How stable is the child?
- What is their heart rate and blood pressure and do they require inotropes to maintain these?
- If they are on inotropes, are they increasing or weaning?
- Do they have a temperature (usually indicative of an infection)?
- Check that their electrolytes and platelets are within the normal range.
- Is the child's overall fluid balance on a positive or negative trend?
- What is their urine output (normal is 1 ml/kg/hour)
- If they are ventilated note the mode of ventilation, tidal volume, pressures and respiratory rate.
- How much oxygen do they require and is this going up or down?
- If appropriate, look at the child's blood gas results with special reference to $pCO_2$.
- Chest X-rays should inform the assessment and treatment options, compare most recent with previous films to determine any new focal problems or changes.

> **Box 1.4** Signs of respiratory distress
>
> Raised respiratory rate (dependent on age)
>
> Subcostal recession
>
> Intercostal recession
>
> Sternal recession
>
> Tracheal tug/head bob
>
> Nasal flare
>
> Grunting (auto PEEP)
>
> Apnoea
>
> Respiratory arrest
>
> Bradycardia
>
> Asystolic cardiac arrest
>
> Death

## Objective assessment

- Colour, pink and well perfused, or are there signs of cyanosis?
- Breathing pattern.
- Adequately undress the child to observe the neck and torso.
- Any signs of respiratory distress (Box 1.4).
- Feel the child's chest movement, any moving secretions palpable? (tactile fremitus).
- Auscultate.
- Suction may be indicated as part of the assessment.
- Finally, establish what the child's main problems are and whether these problems can be addressed by physiotherapy intervention.

The references for this chapter can be found on www.expertconsult.com.

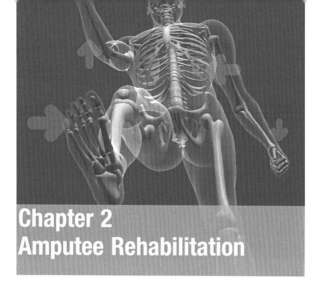

# Chapter 2
# Amputee Rehabilitation

## Introduction

- Amputation is the removal of a limb or part of a limb by surgery or trauma.
- Distinction must be made between those with acquired amputation through surgery or trauma and those with congenital limb deficiency.
- A student or novice physiotherapist who works in amputee rehabilitation will have the opportunity to acquire specific amputee-related knowledge and skills, e.g. oedema control, gait analysis and re-education and prosthetic management. Additionally they will be able to apply and develop musculoskeletal knowledge alongside communication skills, problem-solving and multidisciplinary team (MDT) working.
- The student or novice physiotherapist may assess and treat the primary amputee and/or the established amputee (LLIC 2010).
- Where there is no on-site specialist physiotherapist available for supervision and guidance it is important for the therapist to know when and where to seek specialist support, e.g. via a regional prosthetic centre.
- This chapter will cover the assessment of the adult amputee with acquired lower limb amputation, with some reference to the adult upper limb amputee.
- Advice on the assessment of the child with acquired amputation or congenital absence should be sought from regional specialist centres.

### Amputations, a brief history

- Amputations have been carried out throughout history and until the advent of anaesthesia, improved surgical techniques, control of blood loss and effective infection control in the 19th century the mortality rate amongst amputees was high.

- The history of prosthetics can be traced back to 1000 BC, with manufacturing and function remaining basic until the 16th century.
- Throughout history warfare has resulted in accelerated prosthetic developments. Materials, design, function and patient comfort have evolved and been refined as technology has advanced (Bowker and Pritham 2004).

## Causes of amputation

- Current demographic data are based on amputees referred to specialist prosthetic rehabilitation centres (Limbless-statistics, 2012).
- Currently there are no national data for all amputations performed in the UK, nevertheless it is estimated that a small number of primary amputees are not referred for prosthetic rehabilitation including amputees who have been assessed by health professionals where prosthetic mobility is considered unsafe or inappropriate.
- In some cases amputees choose not to achieve prosthetic mobility, irrespective of ability.

Consequently, according to Limbless-statistics, 2012 approximately 5000 amputations are performed annually in the UK and referred for assessment for prosthetic rehabilitation, with over 90% of these being lower limb (LL).

## Context, United Kingdom

- The number of persons with amputation (the amputee) in the UK – 62000 (Limbless-statistics, 2012) – is small relative to the total population, i.e. approximately 9 per 100000, in comparison to approximately 180 stroke patients (per 100000) (ONS, 1994–1998). The likelihood of every undergraduate student or novice physiotherapist experiencing amputee rehabilitation is therefore small.
- Most amputees receive early rehabilitation as in-patients in an acute hospital setting and form part of a physiotherapist's caseload that includes non-amputee patients. Depending on the cause of amputation the amputee may be managed on a surgical, orthopaedic or care of the elderly ward and this may be for a prolonged period. Exceptions to this are a vascular unit within a hospital or a specialist rehabilitation ward attached to a prosthetic rehabilitation unit in a disability service centre (DSC).
- Physiotherapists are well placed as key health professionals in amputee management since initial contact can be prior to amputation surgery, in the community or later in the care pathway at review and follow up of the 'established' amputee. Irrespective of the setting, guidelines recommend that physiotherapists specialised in amputee rehabilitation be responsible for the physiotherapy management of amputees (Broomhead et al 2003, 2006). A holistic multidisciplinary approach is advocated at all stages of rehabilitation from pre-operative assessment through to prosthetic discharge (Broomhead et al 2003, 2006). At all stages patients' and carers' wishes must be considered.
- Following amputation the common goal for most amputees is to achieve functional independence, ideally using a prosthesis. Amputees face many challenges, particularly physical and psychosocial ones which can change with age and acquired conditions affecting potential for rehabilitation, mobility and overall function (Schoppen et al 2003). Physiotherapy assessment is indicated at several stages during rehabilitation and at further and often unrelated times during the life of an amputee.

# Assessment

## Preoperative physiotherapy assessment

- Recommended where practicable, as this provides an opportunity to observe and note joint contractures, muscle weakness or gait deviations, often present if a patient has had a prolonged period of pain and immobility.

- The physiotherapist can demonstrate equipment, advise on exercises to reduce and/or prevent weakness and prevent contractures.

- Information gained from assessment can be shared with medical colleagues to facilitate the decision process regarding level of amputation and early post-operative management.

- This assessment also offers the potential amputee the opportunity to discuss any concerns and ask questions.

## Postoperative physiotherapy assessment

- Usually performed routinely postoperatively, preprosthetically, as part of prosthetic rehabilitation, as part of prosthetic review or following further amputation surgery or acquired pathology.

- Aspects of the assessment are similar to other areas within a physiotherapist's scope of practice, e.g. an amputee with a musculoskeletal problem would have the same tests performed prior to local soft tissue treatment. An amputee with a neurological condition would have the same assessment of balance, tone and function as performed for a patient managed in a neurological rehabilitation setting.

- The interpretation of physiotherapy assessment defines the goals for treatment, including suitability for prosthetic rehabilitation.

- Ongoing evaluation involving the use of valid, outcome measures, is critical to achieving successful patient outcomes.

## Prosthetic assessment

- Following surgery the majority of amputees are referred for prosthetic rehabilitation at their local DSC of which there are 43 in the UK.

- Most will receive their initial prosthetic treatment at the centre as outpatients and will continue their prosthetic rehabilitation at their local hospital or via community services.

- However not all amputees referred to DSC will be fitted with a prosthesis.

- Physiotherapy assessment findings contribute to the MDT decision regarding an amputee's suitability for this stage of rehabilitation.

# General considerations

## Age

- The incidence of lower limb amputation increases with age. The average age of a patient requiring a first amputation is 69; 28% of all new referrals to prosthetic centres in 2006 were over the age of 75.

- Unlike LL amputees, most UL amputees are in the younger age groups which reflects the aetiology of the condition, i.e. mainly trauma. Three in every five UL referrals were aged between 16 and 54 years (Limbless-statistics, 2012).

## Gender

- The male to female ratio is approximately 3 : 2 (Limbless-statistics, 2012).

## Levels of amputation

- The levels of amputation of the upper and lower limb are shown in Figures 2.1 and 2.2 and the incidence of the amputations at these levels is listed in Box 2.1.

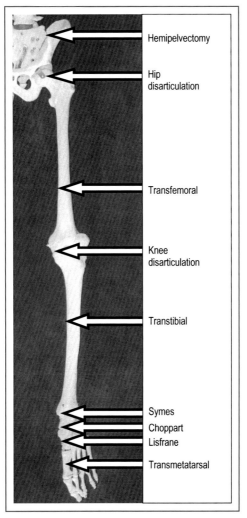

Hemipelvectomy

Hip disarticulation

Transfemoral

Knee disarticulation

Transtibial

Symes

Choppart

Lisfrane

Transmetatarsal

**Figure 2.1 Levels of amputation in the lower limb.**

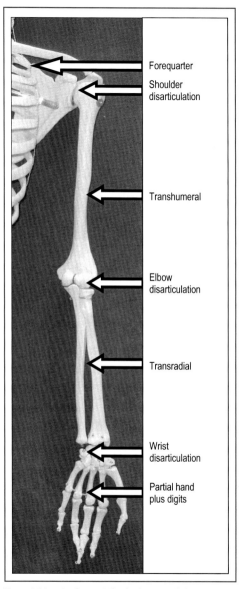

Figure 2.2 Levels of amputation in the upper limb.

Forequarter

Shoulder
disarticulation

Transhumeral

Elbow
disarticulation

Transradial

Wrist
disarticulation

Partial hand
plus digits

> **Box 2.1** Causes and incidence of amputations in the lower and upper limb (Limbless-statistics, 2012)
>
> **Lower Limb (LL)**
> - 72% of LL amputations are caused by dysvascularity e.g. peripheral vascular disease and/ or diabetes.
> - 50% of patients with vascular disease have diabetes and account for a third of patients referred for prosthetic rehabilitation.
> - Other causes of LL amputation include:
> - 7% Trauma e.g. RTA, conflict
> - 3% Neoplasia
> - 8% Infection e.g. meningococcal septicaemia
> - 3% Congenital deformity
> - 9% Other causes or no cause provided
>
> **Upper Limb (UL)**
> - Patients with (UL) amputation account for only 5% of the total amputee population, and the cause is mostly traumatic (53% of cases).
> - Other causes of UL amputation include:
> - 11% Dyvascularity
> - 10% Neoplasia
> - 6% Infection
> - 1% Neurological disorder
> - 20% Other or no cause provided
> - Congenital deformity accounts for approximately 3% of all patients with limb absence
> - A total of 4,574 lower limb and 215 upper limb amputations were recorded in the United Kingdom in 2006/07.

## Mortality

- Perioperative mortality rates are related to level of amputation, cause of amputation, age and co-morbidities (Engstrom and Van de Ven 1999).
- Recent figures from the Vascular Society of Great Britain quote a perioperative mortality rate ranging from 10% in transtibial amputees to 24% at transfemoral level.
- Data indicate 50–60% survival at 2 years and 30–40% at 5 years (vascular cause of amputation).

## Additional information to consider

- Anatomy of the lower and upper limbs
- Vascular system
- Pathology of causes of amputation, associated conditions and complications including:
- Peripheral vascular disease (PVD)
- Cerebrovascular accidents
- Myocardial infarction
- Mesenteric (gut) infarction

- Diabetic retinopathy and visual impairment
- Diabetic neuropathy in hands and feet
- Renal disease
- Additional trauma or associated injuries, e.g. burns, blast, compression
- Elective amputation following trauma, e.g. following reconstructive orthopaedic management
- Specific investigations prior to amputation surgery:
- Segmental pressure monitoring – uses pressure gradients to determine blood flow
- Colour Doppler ultrasound – measures velocity of blood flow. Increased velocity indicates narrowing, zero velocity indicates occlusion
- Magnetic resonance angiography
- Angiography – use of injected contrast agent into artery (usually femoral) to enable imaging of vasculature to identify extent and level of vascular insufficiency to determine either further intervention or level of amputation
- Examples of vascular intervention (Beard et al 2009)
- Depending on the location and extent of the vascular disease the following may be options
- Surgical or chemical sympathectomy
- Angioplasty
- Stenting
- Embolectomy
- Bypass grafts, e.g. femoral popliteal
- Amputation surgical techniques (Smith et al 2004), e.g.
- The long posterior flap and skew flap at transtibial level
- Anterior and posterior flap at transfemoral level
- Other investigations include
- X-rays – can assist with decisions regarding level and length of amputation
- Biopsy – tumour
- Pain – causes and influencing factors include, infection, joint pain, psychological (Engstrom & Van de Ven 1999; Ehde et al 2000; Hanley et al 2004, 2006)
- Gait, i.e. normal gait (Whittle 2007)
- Grieving process (Fischer 2009)
- Multidisciplinary team approach (Ham et al 1987; Stewart & Jain 1993; Pernot et al 1997)
- Prosthetics, i.e. basic examples and fit of prosthesis (Smith et al 2004).

## Considerations immediately prior to undertaking an assessment

- Therapeutic setting.
- Type of surgical anaesthesia used – general versus spinal or chemical block.
- Primary or established amputee.
- Timing, e.g. postoperative, preprosthetic or prosthetic stage of rehabilitation, prosthetic review.

- Pain control. Ensuring that pain is adequately controlled will enable the amputee to engage effectively in the assessment process and allow the therapist to perform a thorough and accurate assessment.
- Therapy/MDT assessment approach, i.e. profession-specific or joint assessment (e.g. OT and PT). Joint assessments reduce repetition for the amputee and can enrich the quality of the information obtained.
- Next of kin and/or carers. In some instances it is necessary to seek permission from others, e.g. for children, vulnerable adults.
- Awareness of prior or associated assessments.
- Access to existing reports, e.g. home access visit. These can help target assessment questions.
- Environment, e.g. gym setting with adjustable plinth, ward and hospital bed, home.
- Patient to be suitably dressed for assessment.
- Removal of footwear to allow inspection of remaining foot.
- Acknowledge cause and associated physical problems, e.g. neural damage or fractures.
- Awareness of feelings of anxiety and loss, sadness and sometimes depression. There may be associated family or personal loss. In cases of severe trauma some amputees may experience post traumatic stress disorder (PTSD).
- Early identification of cognitive problems will influence the extent of assessment, goal setting, treatment plan and outcomes of rehabilitation. If not performing a joint assessment early referral to an occupational therapist or psychologist may be required.

## Where to find important information

- Patient medical notes, current and past
- Prosthetic file in DSCs
- Reports/correspondence from referring colleagues, e.g. GP referral, home visit reports, social worker report, district nurse, school (e.g. paediatric amputee)
- Members of the amputee MDT
- Patient
- Next of kin/parents/carers.

## Subjective assessment

- The approach will be similar to history taking in any of the core assessments.

### Age and gender

### History of present condition

- Date of amputation, cause and level
- History of investigations/surgery prior to amputation
- Mobility, function and social participation prior to amputation
- Co-morbidities and concurrent pathologies/injuries.

## Past and relevant medical history

- Diabetes – diabetic control and management, previous healing rates; presence of diabetic peripheral neuropathy and/or glaucoma, renal disease.
- PVD – presence and manifestation of intermittent claudication; effects on remaining limb.
- Osteoarthritis – limitations of movement, joint replacement affecting pre-amputation mobility.
- Rheumatoid arthritis – active/burnt out; joint deformities; hand function will be important for ability to transfer and don a prosthesis.
- CVA – important factor in determining level of amputation and likely outcomes.
- THREAD (*T*hyroid disorders, *H*eart problems, *R*heumatoid arthritis, *E*pilepsy, *A*sthma or other respiratory problems, *D*iabetes).
- General health, e.g. recent weight loss/gain.
- Previous surgical history, e.g. vascular/orthopaedic reconstructive surgery, other amputation surgery or general surgery.
- Smoking/alcohol history.
- Vision.
- Hearing.

## Drug history

- Current medication. Awareness of impact of specific medications on wound healing, exercise tolerance, mood, e.g. steroids, anticoagulants, diuretics, use of GTN, antidepressants
- Pain control, i.e. residual limb and/or phantom limb pain/other
- Allergies (e.g. dressings).

## Psychosocial history

- This may be done in conjunction with occupational therapy colleagues
- Home, e.g. accommodation, flat, house, stairs
- Owner/rented accommodation
- Occupation/financial situation, e.g. in need of advice regards entitlements and benefits
- Interests and hobbies
- Social support, i.e. family members, neighbours, community
- Driving and transport
- Pre-amputation level of mobility and function, e.g. premorbid use of walking aids
- Cognition
- Mood/motivation/mental health status, presentation, e.g. posture, willingness to engage with history taking and assessment process.

## Pain history

- Back and/or neck pain
- Joint pain
- Neuropathic pain
- Other

- Amputees will routinely experience postoperative residual limb discomfort or pain (RLP)
- Amputees can also experience phantom limb sensation (PLS) which may be painful (PLP)
- Chronic residual limb pain is pain that continues for more than 6 months post amputation
- An amputee's response to pain can indicate acceptance or otherwise of amputation, adjustment to altered body image.

## Objective assessment

### Range of movement (ROM)

- Limited ROM (both UL and LL) will influence rehabilitation outcomes.
- Existing and presenting deformities and/or unstable joints proximal to the residuum and in the remaining limb will influence the potential for prosthetic use and mobility.
- The most common joint contracture (which may be 'fixed' or reversible) for transfemoral amputees is hip flexion, abduction and external rotation (Figure 2.3).
- Fixed flexion contracture deformity of greater than 25° can impact on prosthetic comfort, prosthetic prescription, mobility and energy expenditure.
- Flexion deformity of the knee in the transtibial amputee will influence prosthetic fitting, gait and function.
- It should be noted that skilled prosthetists and prosthetic technicians can modify a prosthesis to accommodate some degree of fixed flexion deformity and/or contracture.
- Prosthetic prescription can also accommodate some instability of the knee joint.
- Limited ROM in the upper limbs may compromise ability to perform activities of daily living (ADLs), transfers and restrict wheelchair mobility.

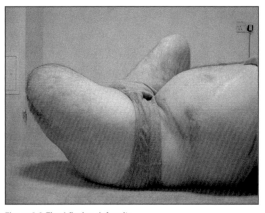

**Figure 2.3 Fixed flexion deformity.**

## Muscle strength

- A grade less of than 4 (Oxford Scale Grading) (Medical Research Council 1976) in all major muscle groups in the upper and lower limb can influence the amputee's ability to achieve functional independence, e.g. to carry out ADLs, self propel a wheelchair, administer wheelchair brakes, transfer independently, and to stand from sitting and to walk.
- Weakness in the LLs will contribute to gait deviations.

## Balance and co-ordination

- Poor balance and righting reactions may compromise mobility and function in terms of safety and is associated with an increased risk of falls.
- An inability to safely reach outside base of support will hinder functional tasks, e.g. to operate footplates, dress and undress and to transfer.

## Proprioception

- This is dependent on amputation level, i.e. the higher the level the greater the loss of proprioception and balance influencing mobility, function and safety.

## Comorbidities

- The presence of comorbidities, e.g. CVA, fracture, will influence the objective assessment and may indicate further specific therapy assessment. Comorbidities will affect treatment planning and outcomes.

## Sensation

- Testing sensation of the remaining lower leg and residuum is especially important for those amputees at risk of peripheral neuropathy, i.e. the amputee with PVD and/or diabetes (Potter et al 1998) (Figure 2.4).
- The amputee should be able to report any pressure or shear forces on vulnerable tissue areas on the residual limb and on the toes, metatarsal heads and heels of the remaining limb.
- Unreported and unresolved adverse pressure will result in the breakdown of skin and soft tissue that may develop into ulcers and delay the achievement of functional outcomes.

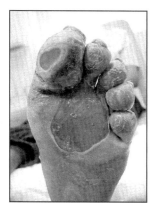

**Figure 2.4 Ulcerated diabetic foot.**
*Reprinted from Foster A 2006, Podiatric assessment and management of the diabetic foot, published by Churchill Livingstone, with permission from Elsevier Ltd.*

## Pain

- Pain after amputation is common.
- The amputee may report RLP or PLP; however, phantom sensation can be painless.
- The presence of pain may influence the amputee's ability to engage in rehabilitation.
- Occasionally pain can become a long-standing problem.
- Objective measures to assess and evaluate RLP and PLP include visual analogue scales (VAS) and body charts (Fox and Day 2009).
- Palpation of the residual limb, e.g. for neuroma, and the assessment of ROM in proximal joints, including neck and back can assist in the diagnosis and management of RLP, PLP and/or coexisting pain presentations.

## Prosthetic function and gait

- If the amputee is a prosthetic user the fit and alignment of the prosthesis must be assessed along with observational gait analysis.
- This aspect of assessment is likely to take place at prosthetic review, in anticipation of a new prosthetic prescription, due to additional pathology or following a fall.
- Additionally a range of incidents can prompt a referral (patient self referral, or via the MDT) to physiotherapy, e.g. loss of confidence, deteriorating ability to walk or perform functional activities or the onset of pain.
- Prior to observing and assessing amputee gait, routine aspects of assessment should be conducted and noted as findings may indicate the cause of gait deviations and/or difficulties.
- Prosthetic function and gait assessment include observing the prosthetic donning procedure, the fit of the prosthesis and routine functional activities such as sit to stand, walking (Figure 2.5) and stairs.
- Walking aids required must be noted along with apparent confidence and balance.

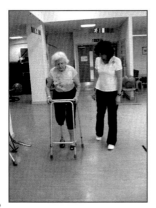

**Figure 2.5 Gait observation.**

- The use of validated outcome measures should be incorporated into this assessment to provide objective benchmarking, e.g. Houghton scale, Timed Up and Go, Activities-specific Balance Confidence Scale – UK (ABC-UK) (BACPAR 2010, Condie et al 2006).

## Other considerations and observations

### The residual limb

- Skin colour and condition, e.g. in the dysvascular amputee the colour of the residuum may be dusky, red or white and fragile. The residuum may be cool in temperature with poor vascular refill (i.e. blanching on pressure with slow return to normal skin colour). Skin may be thin and shiny with minimal or no hair growth. These observations, the presence of ulcers or a non-healing amputation wound, are indicators of poor vascularity and vulnerability to skin or wound breakdown.
- The presence of infection will compromise wound healing and predispose to tethered or adherent scarring affecting successful prosthetic fitting.
- Delayed wound healing will lengthen the period for rehabilitation and can affect the amputee's mood and motivation.
- Scarring, skin grafts or poor sensation will influence prosthetic prescription, mobility and function.
- Signs of skin irritation can indicate reaction to dressings, stump socks, prosthetic materials or poor personal hygiene.
- The shape and length of the residuum, the position of suture lines and scars, proximal joint deformities and/or bony prominences will impact on prosthetic socket shape and design, comfort and mobility.
- Oedema is a normal response to amputation surgery. Its control, reduction and evaluation will influence the progression of rehabilitation.

### The remaining leg

- The same factors that relate to the vascularity of the residuum relate to the remaining leg and provide an indication of the viability, potential for weight bearing required for transfers and walking, and long-term outcome.
- The overall condition of the foot, e.g. joint, bone and/or skin changes, sensation, and the presence of suitable protective covering and footwear, are important factors for function and prosthetic mobility.
- Care of the remaining leg forms an important part of treatment (Figure 2.6).

### Cardiovascular (CV) and respiratory systems

- Prosthetic mobility demands an increase in energy expenditure and a need for increased exercise tolerance.
- Transfemoral amputees use more energy to walk than normals (Waters and Mulroy 2004).
- The prevalence of coexisting cardiovascular and/or respiratory disease in patients with dysvascular amputation is high and comorbid heart disease may prevent functional independence (Roth et al 1998).
- An ability to use a wheelchair and early walking aid (EWA) such as the pneumatic post-amputation mobility aid (PPAM Aid) can indicate capacity to meet an increased energy demand.

AMPUTEE REHABILITATION

2

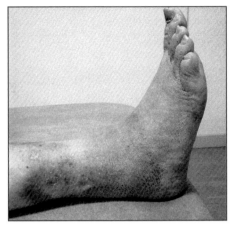

**Figure 2.6 The remaining limb.**

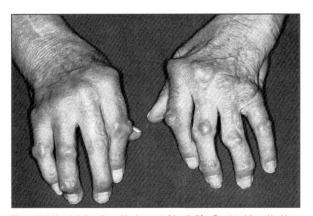

**Figure 2.7 Hand deformity with rheumatoid arthritis.** *Reprinted from Hochberg MC 2003 Rheumatology, 3rd edition, published by Churchill Livingstone, with permission from Elsevier Ltd.*

### Postural and facial characteristics

- Postural and/or facial effects may be indicative of pain, apprehension or depression, e.g. postural kyphosis may reflect an amputee's low psychological status with regard to acceptance of their loss and ability to engage in the assessment process.

### Hand dexterity

- Poor hand dexterity (e.g. rheumatoid arthritis) will affect ADLs such as dressing, and the ability to donn and doff a prosthesis (Figure 2.7 – refer to Chapter 15 for more detail).

## Functional assessment of personal ADLs

- This provides information about the amputee's physical ability to carry out routine functional tasks, cognitive ability to problem-solve and learn new tasks – simple and more complex – and capacity to remember and retain information.
- These abilities contribute to the assessment for suitability for prosthetic mobility.
- Examples of ADLs include:
- Transfers
- Bed mobility
- Ability to manoeuvre wheelchair
- Independence with washing, dressing and eating.

## Prosthetic referral

- Not every amputee is suitable for prosthetic rehabilitation and this is common with the older transfemoral amputee.
- There is a low success rate in terms of prosthetic function in the older amputee (Cumming et al 2006; Callaghan and Condie 2004; Davies and Datta 2003).
- It should be noted that if a decision is made not to refer a patient for prosthetic rehabilitation (by either the amputee or the MDT) this should be reviewed where circumstances change physically or psychosocially.
- Independent and safe wheelchair mobility is a positive outcome for many amputees and an important goal for physiotherapy treatment.
- To assist the decision-making process with respect to assessing an amputee's suitability for using a prosthesis, functionally and safely, there are some broad guidance criteria:
- The residual limb wound should be healing – an unhealed wound is not a contraindication to prosthetic mobility, but may compromise prosthetic prescription
- The amputee must be able to understand and remember instructions. This relates to safety and also the capacity for problem-solving and reasoning
- The amputee must demonstrate independent transfers to and from a wheelchair – indicating safe ability to achieve independence with ADLs
- Independent wheelchair mobility indoors – as above
- The amputee must be able to push up from sitting to standing independently within parallel bars and maintain independent standing (with assistance of parallel bars) – this indicates levels of strength, endurance and balance
- Wound healing permitting, the patient should be able to mobilise with an EWA, this challenges strength, balance, co-ordination and cardiovascular tolerance (see Condie et al 2011, Gailey et al 2002).

## Additional specific factors that may influence prosthetic referral include

- A hip or knee flexion deformity greater than 25° can compromise prosthetic fit, comfort and stability.
- Hand dexterity required to don and doff prosthesis independently.
- Ability to wash and dress independently.
- Motivation, i.e. does the amputee want to walk?

- Does the amputee appreciate what is involved to achieve safe prosthetic mobility?
- Comorbidities.
- A premorbid history of falls.
- Poor social support.

---

**Tip!**

Where a prosthesis will not assist a transfemoral amputee to transfer, a prosthesis can facilitate the transfer process in the case of the single transtibial amputee.

---

## Objective testing

### ROM and strength

- Assessment will follow that of a MSK physical assessment using goniometry and the MRC scale.
- Thomas's test is particularly important for assessing the true extent of hip flexion contracture (Figure 2.8).
- Observation of muscle wasting and tone will be an indicator of weakness, inhibiting pain or long-standing immobility.

### Balance

- Formal validated tests for balance, e.g. Berg balance/TUAG/180° Turn test are not possible in the primary amputee without a prosthesis (Berg et al 1995).
- Functional Reach Test/Measure of Quads strength are objective measures of balance and risk of falls (Campbell et al 1997).

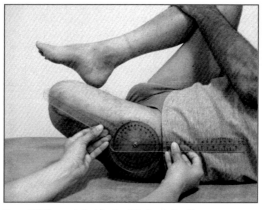

**Figure 2.8 Thomas's test for fixed flexion deformity.**

> **Tip!**
>
> An amputee's ability to move out of base of support, e.g. bend down to take off footwear or remove clothing from bottom half are good indicators of dynamic balance.

## Sensation/proprioception

- Use of differentiation testing, e.g. temperature, light touch, pin prick are all useful tests for assessing general sensation both on the residuum and remaining leg.
- For more in-depth assessment of the diabetic foot the use of a monofilament can provide useful evidence.
- Discernment of 10 points out of 10 is tested – failure to discern all 10 would indicate a foot at risk of being unable to detect pain or pressure and therefore at risk of ulceration and tissue breakdown (Abbott et al 2002).

> **Tip!**
>
> The inability to approximate the palmar surfaces, or make the 'Prayer' sign, can demonstrate limited joint mobility in other joints, e.g. the foot. This in turn can lead to increased pressures on the plantar aspect of the foot and if combined with a neuropathy can lead to ulceration (Goldsmith et al 2002).

## Pain

- The nature and pattern of pain must be recorded. Questioning of pain presentation includes:
- Residual limb or phantom
- Distribution
- Description, e.g. burning, stabbing, drawing, pins and needles, intermittent, constant
- Intensity (VAS) and pattern over 24-hour period
- Triggers, i.e. easing and aggravating factors, e.g. medications, exercise
- Impact on socialisation and participation.

## Additional assessment considerations for the bilateral amputee

### HPC

- The reported long-term prognosis for single vascular amputees is the likelihood of losing the remaining leg within 3 years (Gonzales et al 1974).
- Mortality rates rise after 5 years following the first amputation (Engstrom and Van de Ven 1999).
- Whether the amputee has previously been a single amputee or has become a bilateral as a primary will be significant in their overall management.
- If originally a single amputee their outcome as a prosthetic user will be an important factor in assessment, subsequent treatment planning and potential outcome as a prosthetic user.

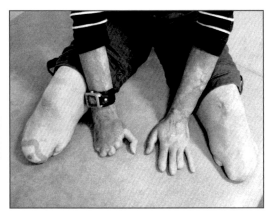

**Figure 2.9 Complex trauma with multiple limb loss.**

### Energy expenditure

- Study findings vary in relation to actual figures of the increase in energy expenditure for walking, but the overall consensus shows an increase in energy cost as levels become higher (Waters and Mulroy 2004).

### ROM

- The importance of maintaining hip and knee extension needs to be emphasised with the bilateral amputee in relation to facilitating transfers and for mobility.

### Balance

- This is critical for a bilateral amputee's ability to transfer safely and independently for functional tasks, e.g. toilet transfers.
- Static and dynamic sitting balance must be assessed on varying surfaces, including low air-loss mattress and gym plinth.
- The more proximal the amputation the greater the loss of stability and challenge to balance.

### UL and trunk strength

- The bilateral amputee will be reliant on good UL and trunk strength to enable independent transfers and self-propulsion in a wheelchair.

### Complex trauma

- The combination of UL with LL loss will influence the assessment approach and the prioritisation of treatment interventions (Figure 2.9).

## Assessment considerations for the UL amputee

### HPC

- The most common cause of amputation in the UL amputee is trauma. Amputation may happen as part of the trauma itself.
- In some cases where limb salvage and reconstructive surgery have not achieved a successful outcome, elective amputation may be performed, e.g. where

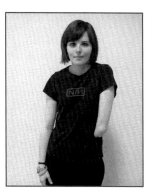

**Figure 2.10 Upper limb amputee posture.**

trauma is associated with a totally avulsed brachial plexus amputation, may be a choice where the arm remains flail and insensate.

- Patients with amputations as a result of infection (e.g. meningococcal septicaemia) often have multiple amputations involving UL and LL.

## ROM, muscle strength, balance and proprioception

- The cervical and thoracic spines, the shoulder girdle and all joints proximal to amputation level in both arms should be assessed.
- In the bilateral UL amputee the neck, hips, knees and feet will be used in ADLs and therefore must be included in assessment.
- Restricted movement and strength will limit function, predispose to postural and gait deviations, affect balance, may contribute to discomfort or pain and will influence function and effective prosthetic use.

## Observation of posture and gait

- The most common postural deviations observed in the UL amputee are internal rotation and adduction of the glenohumeral joint, restricted cervical rotation and side flexion, reduced arm swing in walking accompanied by thoracic side flexion to the amputated side (Figure 2.10).

## Hand dominance. Functional assessment of ADLs

- In the case of the single UL amputee the remaining arm will become the dominant arm.
- Dexterity and ability to perform functional tasks must be assessed.

## Pain

- The presence of discomfort or pain in either arm will influence independence with functional activities and prosthetic use.
- Pain in the remaining arm may be caused by overuse following initial trauma or amputation.

## Psychological factors

- The loss of an arm has considerable psychological consequences.
- The hand is a significant factor in body image, personality, independence and livelihood (Carnegie 1999).

## Treatment planning for the amputee

- A problem list and treatment plan, including agreed achievable goals, should be formulated in partnership with the patient (Broomhead et al 2006).

- Using a tool such as the International Classification of Functioning, Disability and Health (ICF 2010) model can assist the evaluation of the assessment findings (Geertzen 2008).

- The impact of physical, personal, social and environmental factors will influence the reality of attainable rehabilitation goals and will guide the treatment plan.

- Considering these together with assessment findings the physiotherapist can identify the amputee's main problems, discuss, agree and set goals to prioritise treatment planning.

- It is recommended that the 'SOAP' format is used for recording treatment.

The references for this chapter can be found on www.expertconsult.com.

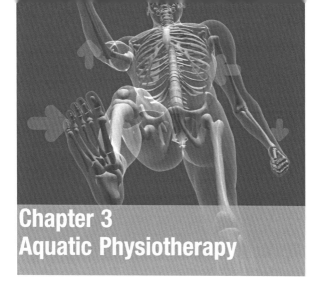

# Chapter 3
# Aquatic Physiotherapy

## Introduction

- Aquatic physiotherapy, despite perhaps being the most ancient therapy, is also a contemporary therapy for the modern world.

- A five-year plan published by the Government encompassing the period 2010–2015 emphasises the need for a more preventative, people-centred and productive National Health Service (DOH 2009).

- Modern aquatic physiotherapy involves people who otherwise are likely to be inactive or not regularly involved in exercise (Jackson et al 2004), is suitable for all (Epps 2009), focuses on the individual and can be exceptionally cost-effective (HyDAT, 2009, Maynard 2003).

- Thus aquatic physiotherapy can be argued to be extremely relevant to the future delivery of an efficient and effective health care service.

- Historically, early religious practices in many cultures emphasised the healing powers of water, for example, the Babylonians, the early Hebrews, and ancient Indians.

- The Greco-Roman civilisation made many claims of water treatment and the Romans centred their social lives on their baths. The collapse of the Roman Empire led to a decline in medical and social bathing.

- Immersion in water re-emerged briefly in the Middle Ages in Europe and then again in the 17th century in England (Alder 1983).

- By the mid 20th century many British doctors rejected spa treatment as being unscientific, but it continued to thrive in much of Europe (Kersley 1982).

- Despite the negative opinions of some regarding the benefits of water-borne treatment, from the 1930s onwards the Chartered Society of Physiotherapy (CSP), with the support of rheumatologists, began to train physiotherapists to use water baths as a treatment for rheumatism (Skinner and Thompson 1983).

- This was the beginning of modern aquatic physiotherapy, which can be defined as:

  *'A physiotherapy programme utilising the properties of water, designed by a suitably qualified physiotherapist. The programme should be specific for an individual to maximise function, which can be physical, physiological, or psycho-social. Treatments should be carried out by appropriately trained personnel, ideally in a purpose built, and heated Aquatic Physiotherapy pool' (ATACP 2009).*

- Thus in contemporary health care provision aquatic physiotherapy should form an integral part of a rehabilitation programme and more broadly be considered as a part of the patient pathway.

- It may be used as the only form of treatment being offered at that time, or may form part an overall treatment plan, designed to be complementary to other aspects of a person's planned treatment programme.

- Aquatic physiotherapy is often considered when all other forms of medical and physiotherapeutic intervention have failed.

- During the initial assessment of a patient consideration should be given to the inclusion of aquatic physiotherapy as a primary option in the management of a wide variety of conditions.

- Modern therapists need knowledge and skills to use this treatment safely and effectively (ATACP 2006). To ensure this, the ATACP run a foundation programme for chartered physiotherapists (ATACP 2010).

## Assessment

- The main aspects of the assessment for aquatic physiotherapy are the same as many of the specialist areas within the physiotherapy scope of practice. For example a patient being assessed for a musculoskeletal problem would have the same tests performed for aquatic therapy as would be carried out prior to local soft tissue treatment, exercise or advice on land.

- A patient with a neurological condition would have the same assessment of balance, tone or function as they would prior to land treatment.

- It is recommended that the 'SOAP' note-keeping format is used, and that outcome measures appropriate to the condition are utilised.

- As an alternative the 'Measure it Yourself Medical Outcome Profile' (MYMOP) has the advantage of being non-condition-specific and easily used for most patient groups. It is commonly used outcome measure across aquatic physiotherapy services in the United Kingdom (Paterson 1996).

- It is important to clinically reason why treatment in the pool should be the treatment of choice. Ask the question 'Why water?' (Can the patient be treated more effectively, more easily, or more appropriately in water than on dry land?).

- Without a sound knowledge of the physical properties of water, and the skills to utilise those properties to create effective treatment techniques this question is difficult to answer.

- A part of this chapter concentrates on the relevant physical properties, to assist the reader to be able to form reasoned decisions in this area.

- Knowledge of how a patient's body build or presenting condition can alter their behaviour in water is also vital.

- It is also important to have a clear understanding of the physiological changes that occur when a human body is immersed in water, as these form a large part of the screening process to ensure that the patient is safe to enter the pool.

- In addition, the person's 'confidence' in water needs to be assessed, both prior to and during the initial stages of treatment. Apart from asking the patient if they are happy in water, it is possible to observe clues such as the patient gripping onto the rails tightly, with a marked reluctance to let go, pulling themselves along the rail as they are laid back in water, or a reluctance to put their head or face near the water surface.

## The physical properties of water

- The relevant properties physiotherapists need to be aware of to ensure that patients are appropriately referred and effectively treated in a pool are:
- Hydrostatic pressure
- Relative densities of water compared to other materials
- Buoyancy
- The metacentre
- Turbulence
- Refraction.

## Hydrostatic pressure

- Hydrostatic pressure is created by the weight of water pressing down from above, and acts in all directions at right angles to any solid surface it is in contact with, e.g. the pool walls or patient's body.

- It follows Pascal's principle that this pressure is transmitted equally and undiminished in all directions through any fluid within a confined space (Brody and Geigle 2009).

Pressure = Force / area

i.e. the weight bearing down on a given spot.

- Pressure at the water surface is known as atmospheric pressure and equals 101 kilopascals (kPa).
- Pressure at 1 metre depth = 111 kPa
- Pressure at 2 metre depth = 121 kPa
- Pressure at 10 metre depth = 201 kPa

- In real terms this means that the human body standing in water up to their sternal notch will have a pressure of 120 $g/cm^2$ being exerted on their calf region. This is equivalent to the application of a tight crepe bandage.

- There is 10 times more pressure on the ankles in water at 1 metre depth, than at the water surface.

- The main consideration therapeutically should be in relation to the physiological changes that occur in the patient's body during immersion.

## Density

Density = mass / volume

i.e. the number of molecules in any given space.

## Relative density

- This is the density of any object or substance relative to the same volume of water at 4 °C (the temperature at which water is most dense).
- Water has a density of 1.000 kg/m$^3$ – (l litre of water at 4°C weighs 1 kg).
- The average human body with air in the lungs has a relative density of 0.975, so will float with 2.5% of its volume out of the water (Brody and Geigle 2009).
- This relationship changes throughout life:
  - A baby is less dense (0.860 kg/m$^3$) so will float with 14% of its body out of the water.
  - As muscle bulk increases so the body becomes more dense (0.975 kg/m$^3$).
  - As muscle and bone bulk decreases in later life, so the body becomes less dense again (0.860 kg/m$^3$).
  - Males tend towards greater muscle bulk, so float less readily.
- Salt water has a density of around 1.024 kg/m$^3$, so a body will float with a greater proportion out of the water.
- Anything less dense than water will float, while anything more dense will sink.
- Densities of different substances (kg/m$^3$)

  | | |
  |---|---|
  | Air | 0.00125 |
  | Cork | 0.22 |
  | Wood | 0.75 |
  | Iron | 7.7 |
  | Gold | 19.3 |
  | Body Fat | 0.92 |
  | Muscle | 1.058 |
  | Rib bone | 1.383 |
  | Tooth | 2.24 |

- As can be seen different parts of the body will behave differently in water due to their differing relative densities, the limbs will tend to sink while the trunk will tend to be more buoyant.

## Buoyancy

- This is the 'Upthrust' effect of water acting on a body, and depends on both the relative density of the object, and the hydrostatic pressure forces being exerted upon it.
- It is governed by Archimedes' principle. This states that 'When a body is wholly or partially immersed in a fluid at rest it will experience an apparent weight loss equal to the weight of the fluid displaced.'
- In other words if you get into a pool of water and the water level rises by 1 inch, if you could weigh that inch of water you would know how much apparent weight relief you were experiencing.
- As a guide for a person standing, immersion to the anterior superior iliac spine gives 50% weight relief, to the xiphisternum 70% weight relief and to C7 90% weight relief (Harrison and Bulstrode 1987).

## Stability in water

- An immersed object is subject to two opposing forces
- Gravity acting downwards
- Buoyancy acting upwards.
- The object's shape, distribution of mass, and density determine its stability.
- When the result of all forces acting on a body equal zero; the body is said to be in equilibrium.

## Centre of buoyancy (COB)

- This is the single point in an immersed object around which the buoyancy (upthrust) forces act.
- This point is the centre of gravity of the shape of the displaced fluid (i.e. its centre of gravity), and is therefore not a fixed point.
- This point moves as the attitude of the immersed body changes.
- In a body at rest it is slightly superior and anterior to the centre of gravity.

## Moment of inertia

- A measure of an object's resistance to changes to its rotation.
- Initiation of rotation is harder in objects with a long radius.

## Metacentre (turning forces in water)

- The metacentre is the midpoint at which a body can be held in perfect balance.
- The term 'metacentre' is not really important, but the effects it has are.
- It is the naval term given to the resultant restoring or stabilising torque (twisting force) when the forces of gravity and buoyancy acting on an immersed object are not in the same vertical plane.
- For the human supine in water with arms at the side, the body will be stable side to side (forces of gravity and buoyancy in line).
- Take the right arm out to the side – the centre of gravity (COG) will move to that side, as will the centre of buoyancy (COB). As the arm is relatively dense however (being predominantly bone and muscle), the COG will move further than the COB, so rotational forces will tend to turn the body in that direction.
- If that same arm is lifted out of the water, then the full force of gravity is then imposed on that arm. The COG therefore shifts over to the right, and because there is more 'shape' on the left, the COB moves to that side, the body will turn to the right.
- If the right arm is crossed over the body, then the COG moves to the left, and the COB to the right and the body rolls to the left (Figure 3.1a and b).

## Some factors that alter stability in water

### 'Shape' of the patient

- A person of very slight build will have the centre of buoyancy close to that of the centre of gravity. So in standing will tend to be more stable.

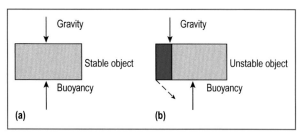

Figure 3.1 (a) Lines of gravity and buoyancy are in line. The object is therefore stable. (b) Line of gravity has shifted to the denser (left hand) end. The object is unstable, and will roll in the direction of the arrows until the opposing forces are once again in line.

- The same applies to the more heavily muscled patient, they will tend to be 'leg heavy' with the legs sinking till they rest on the pool floor.
- A person with a large amount of adipose tissue around the abdomen will have a COG that is higher and more anterior, so they will have a tendency to rock backwards more, with legs that float up more readily.
- A person with physical deformity such as a lateral scoliosis will tend to roll in the water when supine due to the alteration of the position both of the centres of gravity and buoyancy.
- A person with osteoporosis in the lower limbs will float with the legs high, and may even lay with their face immersed when supine unless some sort of buoyancy is applied around the neck/head area.

## Surgery

- Orthopaedic surgery involving the use of metalwork, e.g. a total hip replacement, will make the patient float low on the side of the surgery, due to the greater relative density of the metal compared with the bone it replaces.
- Amputation of a lower limb will tend that patient to float high on the amputated side due to the loss of a relatively dense structure.

## Depth of the water

- Water at S2 level – posture predominantly controlled by gravity.
- Water at T11 level – posture controlled equally by gravity and buoyancy.
- Water at C6/7 – posture predominantly controlled by buoyancy.
- It is more difficult to maintain balance in deeper water, so adopted stable positions facilitate the control of these turning forces, e.g. if you start to topple backwards then tilting the head slightly forwards, or bringing the arms forwards can help to correct the imbalance.

## Hydrodynamics (fluids in motion)

- Hydrodynamics are the effect of movement in water, and largely follow Bernoulli's equation that

Kinetic energy + potential energy + pressure energy = constant

- Even the act of moving through the pool towards your patient will start the water itself moving, and therefore there will be flow.
- There are two types of flow (Brody and Geigle 2009).

## Laminar flow

- This is low velocity, with all the water layers moving at the same speed. The flow is in smooth straight lines and has very little friction with a very small amount of turbulence behind the moving object (and therefore minimal energy loss) (Figure 3.2).

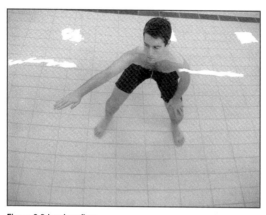

**Figure 3.2 Laminar flow.**

## Turbulent flow

- Potential energy can be assumed to be fixed.
- If kinetic (speed) energy is increased, pressure energy must drop.
- A moving body leaves a wake of disturbed water, this water is swirling (the formation of eddy currents), and therefore moving faster than the still water in front of the body.
- The disturbed area is at a lower pressure and therefore creates a drag to movement (an object will always move from an area of high to an area of low pressure).
- The faster the body moves the greater the wake and the greater the drag effect.
- This is known as turbulence, and causes the greatest resistance to forward movement (Figure 3.3).

## Other factors influencing movement

- A streamlined shape produces less turbulence than a non-streamlined one.
- A bow wave positive pressure created in front of a moving object, impedes forward movement.
- The 'stickiness' of a fluid in motion (water is 790 times 'thicker' than air), i.e. viscosity.

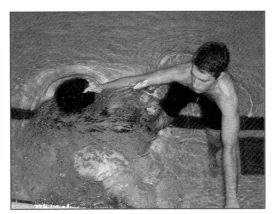

**Figure 3.3 Turbulent flow.**

- Water is adhesive, i.e.: it will stick to an object rather than itself.
- There is a small amount of friction caused as water passes over a moving object.
- The cohesive forces exerted over the surface molecules of a fluid, manifesting itself as an elastic 'skin', i.e. surface tension.

## Refraction

- This is the effect of light rays 'bending' as they pass into a material of a different density.
- Placing a straight rod partly into the water can easily show this, the rod will appear to kink at the water surface (Figure 3.4).

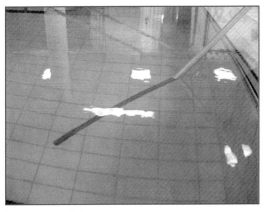

**Figure 3.4 Refraction.**

**Table 3.1** Benefits of aquatic physiotherapy

| Benefit | Reason |
| --- | --- |
| Relief of pain | Warmth of water |
| | Suppression of sns |
| | Stimulation of skin mechanoreceptors |
| Ease of movement | Support offered by buoyancy |
| | Reduced effect of gravity |
| Reduction of spasm | As for pain relief |
| Reduction of oedema | Hydrostatic pressure |
| Resistance to movement | Viscosity of water |
| | Negative drag of turbulence |
| | Weight/density of water |
| | Upward force of buoyancy |
| Enhanced relaxation | Reduced effect of gravity |
| | Support from buoyancy |
| | Reduction in pain |
| | Hypnotic effect of water |
| Enhanced well being | Ability vs disability |
| | Social interaction |
| | Enjoyment |
| Re-education of functional activities | Unencumbered |
| | Support from buoyancy |
| | Resistance to movement |
| | Metacentric effect |
| Enhanced cardiovascular fitness | Resistance to movement |

- The practical effects of this phenomenon to physiotherapists working in a pool environment are:
- Measurements of angle must be taken with the limb completely out of the water
- Submerged items will not be quite where you expect them to be.

## Values and effects of hydrotherapy

- Table 3.1 lists the claimed benefits and effects of aquatic physiotherapy.
- As aquatic physiotherapy is a combination of the effects of immersion and exercise, consideration should also be given to the benefits of exercise alone.
- These have been described as:
- Improved cardiovascular and respiratory function
- Improved neuromuscular and physical performance
- Improved posture and appearance
- Relief of tension
- Stimulation of mental activity
- Increased general feeling of health and well being
- Delaying the ageing process.

## Appropriate use of aquatic therapy

- Aquatic physiotherapy is often considered to be an expensive form of treatment both in terms of staff time and cost of facility.
- It is therefore important to ensure that patients are carefully selected, bearing in mind the following disadvantages unique to this form of treatment:
- Acute fear of water
- Treatment time limitations
- Possible infection spread
- Difficulties isolating some movements
- Patient dependency on treatment
- Contraindications to immersion.
- A common misconception is that aquatic physiotherapy is very expensive. Costing an aquatic physiotherapy service is quite straightforward.
- An average aquatic physiotherapy pool costs around £8.00 per usable hour (2006 costs).
- The following calculation provides an indication of the cost of one 3-hour aquatic physiotherapy session with a band 7 physiotherapist in the pool (2006 costings):

| | |
|---|---|
| 3 Hours Band 7 | £67.92 |
| 3 Hours Band 2 (poolside assistant) | £25.44 |
| 3 Hours Pool time | £23.98 |
| Total | £117.34 |

Average 11 patients treated during the session = cost of £10.66 per treatment

- Comparable costs:

Band 7 physiotherapist carrying out 'normal' outpatient session (3 Hours)

| | |
|---|---|
| 3 Hours Band 7 | £67.92 |
| 0.5 Hours Band 2 | £4.24 |
| Total | £72.16 |

Average 6 patients treated during the session = cost of £12.02 per treatment (Maynard 2003).

- Many of the contraindications to immersion are related to the physiological changes that occur, so a précis of these changes is covered in the following sections.

## The physiology of immersion

- Immersion to the level of the sternum in humans is known as head out of water immersion (HOWI) and causes profound changes physiologically in the body. This chapter intends to look at the changes that occur in the following systems:
- Haematological
- Cardiovascular
- Respiratory
- Renal
- Sympathetic nervous system.

- Knowledge of these changes is critical to ensure safe screening of patients prior to aquatic physiotherapy.

## Haematological and cardiovascular systems

- On entry into water up to the sternal notch, the hydrostatic pressure gradient causes 700 ml of blood to be redirected towards the heart and cardiothoracic compartment from 'blood pooling in the limbs' (Hall et al 1990).
- This increases the central blood volume (CBV), and it is this that triggers many of the physiological changes.
- There is an increase in tissue reabsorption around the capillary networks of the lower limb, as the increased pressure narrows the capillaries and reduces the flow to the venules.
- Venous pressure is reduced, thus increasing the re-absorption force (i.e. the Starling force is tilted towards reabsorption back into the capillaries).
- 'Water immersion causes a haemodilution within the first 30 minutes' (Hall et al 1990).
- With the 700 ml increase in CBV and the haemodilution the following events occur 'immediately immersion is initiated' into thermoneutral water at 33.5–35.5°C (Hall et al 1990):
- 30% increase in cardiac output (Hall et al 1990)
- 50% increase in stroke volume (Weston et al 1987, as cited in Hall et al 1990)
- Reduction in peripheral resistance (Hall et al 1990)
- Blood pressure changes: 'systolic remains unchanged and diastolic drops by about 9 mmHg' (Hall 1996).
- It is important to note that these effects increase as the water temperature rises, so that at 39°C cardiac output increases to 121% (Weston et al 1987).
- Patients with resting angina or uncontrolled cardiac failure should not be taken into the pool due to the increased demand placed on the heart by immersion. Bucking (as cited in Hall 1996) 'recommended that water exercise be avoided for 6 weeks post cardiac event'.
- Also be aware of patients with hypotension, as immersion lowers their diastolic blood pressure still further and they may feel faint or light-headed.

## Respiratory system

- Immersion alters pulmonary function via direct hydrostatic pressure effects on the thorax, cephalad displacement of the diaphragm, and the central hypervolaemia. The following changes take place:
- Expiratory reserve volume decreases (Craig and Dvorak 1975)
- Vital capacity drops by 5–10% (Craig and Ware 1967 as cited in Hall 1990)
- Increase in airway closure (Bondi et al 1976 as cited in Anstey and Roskell 2000)
- Reduced lung compliance largely due to vascular engorgement stiffening the lungs (Dahlback and Lundgren 1972 as cited in Anstey and Roskell 2000)
- 'Tidal volume is not affected' during immersion (Hall 1996).
- Therefore avoid taking patients with shortness of breath at rest (due to a respiratory pathology) into a pool.

- Exercising in water will also increase oxygen consumption compared to exercising on land. 'Oxygen consumption does not increase through warm water immersion per se' (Hall 1996), but when walking on a treadmill in water compared to on land oxygen consumption is 'significantly greater' (Gleim and Nicholas 1989 as cited in Hall et al 1990).
- Therefore oxygen dependency on land can be seen as a relative contraindication.

## Renal system

- Immersion causes an increase in blood flow to the kidneys.
- Kidney metabolism is thus enhanced with greater excretion of sodium and greater urine output.
- Six- to sevenfold increase in urine production (Hall et al 1990)
- Sodium excretion increases by 200–300% (Hall et al 1990, p. 519)
- Atrial natriuretic peptide production doubles (important factor in increased renal output and sodium excretion) (Hall et al 1990, p. 520)
- Antidiuretic hormone and aldosterone production suppressed by stimulation of low-pressure stretch receptors in the atria and pulmonary arteries (Epstein 1976).
- Because of these effects renal failure can be seen as a precaution to immersion in the pool.
- It is essential that patients empty their bladders before getting into the pool, and also that they replenish their fluid loss at the end of the session.

## Sympathetic nervous system

- The sympathetic and parasympathetic nervous systems are part of the autonomic nervous system.
- The sympathetic nervous system activates our fight or flight response and as such is responsible for actions such as increasing our heart rate.
- Thermoneutral HOWI lowers sympathetic activity.
- It acts to 'reduce peripheral vascular resistance to compensate for increases in the stroke volume and cardiac output due to cephalad fluid shift; thus maintaining hemodynamic homeostasis' (Mano 1998)
- By suppressing sympathetic activity it can help reduce neurogenic pain including complex regional pain syndromes (CRPS)
- Schencking et al (2009) found that hydrotherapy was effective at reducing CRPS pain.
- Aquatic therapy may also be responsible for reducing pain because the movement of the water over the skin stimulates mechanoreceptors which in turn closes the pain 'gate' mechanism (Melzack 1981).

## Contraindications and precautions to aquatic physiotherapy (CSP 2006)

### Absolute contraindications

- Acute vomiting or diarrhoea.
- Medical instability following an acute episode such as CVA, DVT, or status asthmaticus, if in doubt then check with the patient's consultant.

- Proven chlorine/bromine allergy.
- Resting angina.
- Shortness of breath at rest.
- Uncontrolled cardiac failure.
- Weight in excess of the evacuation equipment limit of the pool (refer to the local manual handling policy).

## Relative contraindications

- If the following are present aquatic physiotherapy may be considered after a risk-benefit analysis:
- Acute systemic illness/pyrexia
- Irradiated skin due to radiotherapy. Be aware that irradiated skin 'will always be more sensitive to heat' and 'wounds will heal more slowly' (Brooks 1998). Also be aware that chlorine can cause a skin irritation
- Known aneurysm
- Open infected wounds will need to be managed according to local infection control policies
- Poorly controlled epilepsy
- Unstable diabetes and the effects of exercising in the water may result in a patient having an episode of symptoms relating to a drop in their blood sugar. They should be monitored closely for any signs of this occurring and a snack should be available on the pool side
- Thyroid deficiency: 'metabolism of thyroid hormone may be associated with deficient thermoregulation' (Beard et al 1990)
- Patients with neutropenia should not be taken into an aquatic therapy pool when their white blood cell count is very low
- Oxygen dependency.

## Precautions

- Fear of water.
- Behavioural problems.
- Incontinence of urine – patient can be catheterised during session.
- Epilepsy. Clients who suffer from epilepsy can attend aquatic physiotherapy but the epilepsy needs to be controlled by medication such as rectal diazepam which the pool staff need to be trained in administering.
- Haemophilia (check factor VIII or IX) – may need to take clotting factors prior to exercise. Swimming is actually very beneficial for clients with haemophilia (Von Mackensen et al 2009).
- Hypotension.
- Renal failure.
- Widespread MRSA – only as a precaution on poolside as chlorine kills MRSA in the water (Tolba et al 2008).
- Poor skin integrity. e.g. open/surgical wounds.
- Pregnancy if water temperature exceeds 35°C (CSP 2009).
- Contact lenses and conjunctivitis.

- Hearing aids/grommets.
- Impaired vision/sensation/hearing.
- Invasive tubes in situ – PEG sites do not need to be covered.
- Risk of aspiration.
- Incontinence of faeces (less than 2 hourly) – bowel management programme should be established.
- Low calorie intake – 'ensure that aquatic physiotherapy is not used as a means to reduce weight' by drawing up a contract with the client (CSP 2006).
- Prone to blackouts.
- Sickle cell anaemia – swimming in cold water may trigger a painful crisis in some children. 'Cold exposure increases blood viscosity' and can lead to 'even further sickling' (Resar and Oski 1991).
- Inefficient thermoregulation. Be aware that clients can get very cold whilst they are leaving the pool and are still wet. Conversely an aquatic physiotherapy pool room can become very humid in the summer.
- Tracheostomy, current guidelines are being developed. One member of staff is required to look after the tracheostomy and a portable suction machine should be present on the poolside. An appropriately experienced physiotherapist should be present.

The references for this chapter can be found on www.expertconsult.com.

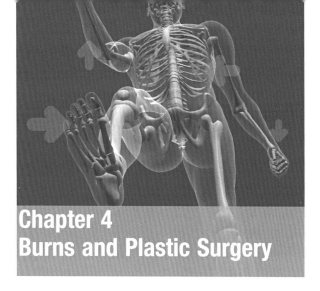

# Chapter 4
# Burns and Plastic Surgery

## Burns

### Introduction

- The assessment and treatment of patients following a burn injury requires management by a dedicated burns team.

- Physiotherapists are an integral part of the team, which also includes; nurses, doctors, plastic surgeons, social workers, dieticians, psychologists and the patient.

- A team approach is regarded as the best way for the assessment and specialist care of these patients as the different role each team member plays contributes to the total care and outcome of the burn patient (Leveridge 1991).

- Injuries depend on the cause and extent of damage, with many being life changing physically, emotionally and psychologically. The injuries also affect the individual's family.

- Management is geared to anticipating potential problems through the assessment of the patient.

- A burn injury comprises of damage to the skin of varying depths and can lead to complete skin loss with or without damage to the underlying tissues. Along with this an individual may present with other signs and symptoms affecting the respiratory, cardiovascular, orthopaedic and neurological systems.

- The depth of skin damage is very important in deciding how the burn will be managed; this is normally conservative management with dressings or management with surgery (Richard and Staley 1994) (Figure 4.1a and 4.1b).

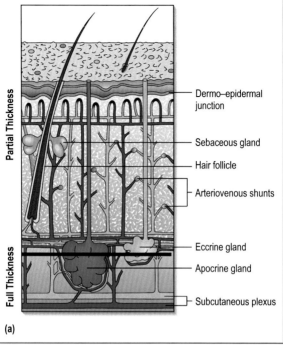

**Figure 4.1a The skin, and damage that occurs following a burn.** *Reprinted from Shamley D 2005, Pathophysiology: an essential text for the allied health professions. Reprinted with permission from Elsevier Ltd.*

## Classification of burns

### Erythema

- The skin appears red, but remains intact.
- This is not documented as part of the burn assessment on a Lund and Browder chart.
- Usually heals within 24–72 hours.

### Superficial burn

- Red appearance, no blister formation, heals in 7 days.
- No residual scarring.

### Partial thickness burn

- Superficial dermal – Tissue damage means leakage of fluid between the layers of epidermis, resulting in blister formation, surrounded by erythema.
- Painful and heals in 10–14 days

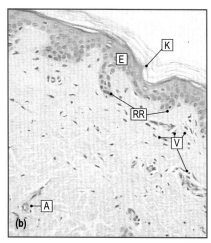

**Figure 4.1b Thick skin.** A. arterioles, V. venules, RR poorly developed rete ridge system, K. keratin layers of thin skin, E. thin epidermal layer.

- Appears red with capillary return
- Forms minimal scarring (Settle 1996).
- Deep dermal – Tissue destruction involves the epidermis and superficial layers of the dermis.
- Appears red without capillary return and no blisters.
- Healing is slow and skin is thin and forms dense scarring (Figure 4.2).

## Full-thickness burn

- These burns are not painful.
- They can involve muscle, tendon and bone.
- Skin loss means that there are no accessory skin structures such as hair follicles to epithelialise.
- Healing will therefore only occur by the epithelium migrating from the edge of the burn wound.
- It is only possible for a very small burn to heal in this way.
- Appears white, waxy looking, or charred black (Figure 4.3).
- Requires management by excision of necrotic tissue and skin grafting (Settle 1996).

## Causes of burns

- Burns can be caused by excessive heat or cold, by chemicals, ultraviolet light or radiation.
- The most common causes of burns requiring hospital treatment are:
- Scalds from hot fluids or steam are common in the under fives and the elderly.

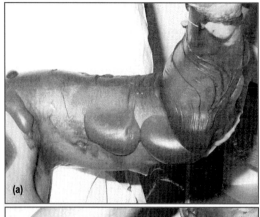

(a)

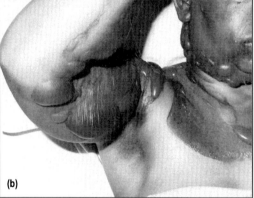

(b)

**Figure 4.2** Partial-thickness dermal burns to both upper limbs and neck with extensive blister formation. *Reprinted from Porter S, 2008, Tidy's physiotherapy, 14th edition. Reprinted with permission from Elsevier Ltd.*

- Explosions, flash flame or steam, bonfires, fireworks, barbeques and the use of flammable liquids such as petrol. Flash burns tend to be partial-thickness burns, but can be deeper if the patient's clothes ignite.
- Flame burns occur when the patient's clothes, hair or skin catch light. The effect of damage from house or car fires is exacerbated by the inhalation of toxic gases from burning household furniture, leading to severe inhalation injuries as well as burns.
- Contact burns from contact with molten metal or plastic are common in industry. An unconscious patient may sustain burns from contact with a cooker or a hot radiator.
- Electrical burns due to electrical current from plugs, sockets and wiring. Deep structures can be involved at the current entry and exit sites on the body. The patient's cardiac status requires close monitoring.

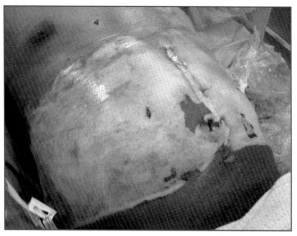

**Figure 4.3** Full-thickness burn of the abdominal region after a fire accident.

- Non-thermal burns, include:
- Chemical damage, acid or alkali substances can cause deep burns, a commonly seen burn is that from contact with cement powder.
- Friction injuries include friction burn from the road surface, e.g. cyclists and motorcyclists.

## History

- Details of how the injury occurred, duration of contact, protection offered by clothing and first aid given can all provide an indication of the type and depth of a burn.
- As burns occur in traumatic circumstances it is important to ensure that other associated traumatic injuries have been eliminated, e.g. fractures, nerve injuries, spinal and head injuries.

## Burns charts

- These are used to record the distribution of the burns and are normally completed by an experienced burns doctor.
- Lund and Browder charts (Figure 4.4) are used to record total body surface area (TBSA) and the depth of the burns, which are documented as partial-thickness (PTB) or full-thickness burns (FTB) (Herndon 2007).
- The larger the total burn surface area, the worse the prognosis for the patient.
- It is important to calculate accurate TBSA, as this will guide the amount of fluid replacement that is required to stabilise the patient.
- The 'rule of nines' is another method of gauging the TBSA. This divides the body surface into 11 areas, each making up 9% of the total, apart from the perineum which is allocated 1% (Porter 2008).

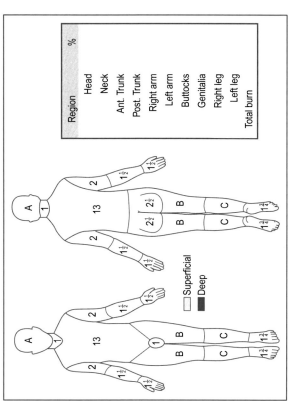

**Figure 4.4** Lund Browder chart.

| Region | % |
|---|---|
| Head | |
| Neck | |
| Ant. Trunk | |
| Post. Trunk | |
| Right arm | |
| Left arm | |
| Buttocks | |
| Genitalia | |
| Right leg | |
| Left leg | |
| Total burn | |

Superficial

Deep

| Table 4.1 Relative percentage of areas affected by growth | | | | | | |
|---|---|---|---|---|---|---|
| Age (years) | 0–1 | 1–4 | 5–9 | 10–14 | 15 | Adult |
| A ½ of head | 9½ | 8½ | 6½ | 5½ | 4½ | 3½ |
| B ½ of one thigh | 2¾ | 3¼ | 4 | 4¼ | 4½ | 4¾ |
| C ½ of one leg | 2½ | 2½ | 2¾ | 3 | 3¼ | 3 |

- There are separate charts for paediatrics. This takes into account the ratio of different body regions to the TBSA, which changes with age (Table 4.1).

## Pathological changes

### Burns shock

- The unique pathological changes include burns shock. This is the inability of the circulatory system to provide oxygen and nutrients and to remove metabolites (Settle 1986).
- The risk of burns shock is due to a decrease in circulatory plasma volume or hypovolaemia caused by plasma leaking from damaged capillaries.
- There is loss of proteins and electrolytes from the blood and there is an increase in blood viscosity.
- The body compensates by shutting down blood supply to the skin, abdominal organs and the kidneys.
- The massive fluid loss and risk of septicaemia gives rise to major cardiovascular instability. If left untreated the fall in cardiac blood pressure can lead to vital organ failure.
- The severity of shock is related to the surface area of skin damage.
- The BP, CVP, haematocrit, urine output and heart rate must be monitored during the acute burn period (Leveridge 1991). Volume of fluid transfusion is adjusted as required to maintain balance.
- The problems of sepsis, massive fluid loss, cardiovascular instability and high airway pressures mean that in order to treat the lung injury, physiotherapists have to repeatedly re-assess the consequences of their treatment in the context of the multi system problems (Keilty 1993).

The symptoms of shock include
- Sweating, cold and pale skin
- Tachycardia
- Hypotension
- Rapid respiratory rate.

Assessment for fluid resuscitation
- Fluid resuscitation will need to be commenced if the TBSA is; >10% in children and >15% in adults (Settle 1996).
- The amount of fluid will need to be calculated, so that it will restore and maintain adequate perfusion of blood to all body tissues. Thirty-six-hour fluid resuscitation is subdivided into numerous periods with the patient being regularly reassessed at the end of each period. Developing signs of shock suggest inadequate fluid management.

- Burns with a TBSA of more than 10% in children and 15% in adults, those with suspected inhalation injury or burns on specific areas of the body, e.g. hands and feet, are generally treated in a specialised burns unit or centre (Porter 2008).

- The specialist burns unit approach leads to improved patient care and provides support for each member of the team in working situations that can be stressful.

- Therapy intervention begins within the first 24–48 hours following admission; therapists have an important role throughout all stages of recovery, to give encouragement, instil confidence and gain co-operation of the patient to enable the patient to be managed effectively.

- Assessment of burns requires good organisational skills, due to the complexity of these injuries.

- The main problems that are likely to be found include:
- Respiratory problems from inhalation burns
- Swelling
- Pain
- Decreased range of movement of involved joints
- Soft tissue contracture
- Scarring
- Loss of function.

- Following admission wounds will be cleaned, debrided and dressed and the process of fluid resuscitation and stabilisation will begin.

- Large burns are life-threatening due to fluid loss, excessive cooling, poorly maintained body temperature and risk of infection.

- Surgeons are responsible for overall evaluation of the burn and patient resuscitation at this stage.

- The therapist will begin their assessment of the patient according to the TBSA of the burn, pre-existing medical conditions and the patient's respiratory status. It is important to confirm details of the injury.

- Information may be obtained from medical notes or charts, other members of the burns team, e.g. doctors, the patient and their family.

- The patient will be nursed in a side room, possibly on an intensive therapy unit (ITU).

- The room temperature is kept higher than normal, at 28°C or more to regulate the patient's subnormal temperature due to burns shock and the loss of the thermoregulation function of the skin, in order to counteract the shutting down of the peripheral circulation.

- There will be strong odours due to plasma leaking from wounds, necrotic tissue and any infections, e.g. Pseudomonas.

- The patient may be ventilated, following an inhalation injury, or if there is excessive head or neck swelling.

- The patient may be sedated or alert and anxious.

- They may have dressed burns and/or exposed burns with associated erythema, blisters, and yellow/white skin, blackened tissues. Dressings may be bulky, to absorb the oozing from wounds.

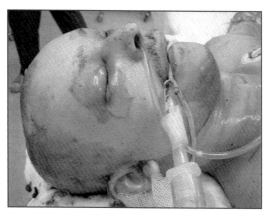

**Figure 4.5** Acute burn showing facial oedema.

- Hands may be in flammazine bags, permitting exercise without the restriction of dressings.
- Swelling may be pronounced, altering facial appearance and possibly reducing vision (Figure 4.5).

## Inhalation injury

- Smoke inhalation is the primary cause of fire-related deaths, increasing mortality by 20% (Shirani et al 1987).
- Inhalation injuries can be due to thermal damage to the upper respiratory tract, or by chemical damage from the inhalation of toxic particles or fumes, such as cyanide.
- The airway responds by producing mucosal oedema, erythema and ulceration.
- The resultant damage affects the body's ability to maintain the ventilation/perfusion balance.
- Secondary damage can occur in response to inflammation, which leads to increased vascular permeability, in turn leading to exacerbation of pulmonary oedema, increasing respiratory resistance and reducing lung compliance.
- Patients with inhalation burns are at risk of developing pneumonia, which can increase the mortality rate by up to 40% (Shirani et al 1987).
- A patient having three of the following clinical factors will in all probability have a significant inhalation injury. These may be difficult to diagnose on first admission. They should be recorded in physiotherapy records.
- Factors indicating an inhalation injury:
- Fire in closed/confined space
- Facial, neck or chest burns and or oedema
- Carbonaceous sputum/bronchial casts
- Perioral burns
- Altered consciousness or confusion
- Respiratory distress

- Hoarse/loss of voice/stridor
- The presence of raised carboxyhaemoglobin in the blood
- Bronchoscopy results showing oedema.
- A patient demonstrating these signs may require intubation and ventilation.
- A respiratory assessment is conducted to determine the treatment needs of the patient, focussing on the patient's ability to maintain a clear airway and should include: respiratory rate, arterial blood gas tensions, degree of cyanosis, chest auscultation and chest radiograph.
- Assessment should include subjective and objective information gathering which is completed and documented within 24 hours of the patient's admission (BASW 2005).
- Pathological changes may not be evident with X-ray in the early stages post burn injury; they may take 24–48 hours to develop.
- Chest problems will often be worsened by multiple surgical procedures required during the acute stage.
- Problems resulting from inhalation injury:
- Reduced chest expansion if burns are over the chest wall
- Sputum retention
- Airway obstruction
- Pneumonia
- Adult respiratory distress syndrome (ARDS).

## Musculoskeletal changes

- The physiotherapist will assess the location of burns, if a burn crosses a joint there is a risk of scar formation, which will lead to contracture.
- All joint ranges will need to be assessed, with the aim of maintaining joint range and soft tissue length to prevent contractures.
- Joint range should be assessed actively if possible and passively, with the degrees of movement being recorded, using goniometry.
- Assessment of muscle power, strength and function should include, where possible, mobility and gait.
- Functional assessment should include the ability to perform activities of daily living (ADL) at home, work roles and any hobbies.
- Assessment may require a dressing to be taken down, if they are restricting movement, limitations may also be due to burnt tissues or the patient's tolerance of pain.
- Pain levels must be assessed and recorded, e.g. using a visual analogue scale (VAS).
- At all stages the therapist should ensure that the patient has adequate pain control and must assess with this in mind.
- Continual reassessment of ROM is required as healing occurs.
- If initial assessment is delayed, it becomes more difficult to assess the patient's potential due to the increased prevalence of oedema at 24–48 hours post burn.
- Oedema is the accumulation of protein-rich fluid or exudate leaking out of injured capillaries, which results from the movement of fluid from intravascular sources to the interstitium through open wounds. This oedema results in a

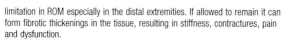

limitation in ROM especially in the distal extremities. If allowed to remain it can form fibrotic thickenings in the tissue, resulting in stiffness, contractures, pain and dysfunction.

- Assessment will need to establish the need for splintage, to position joints and maintain joint range especially in the wrists, hand and elbows.

- Assessment of the burnt hand posture is needed to prevent the development of deformities, e.g. boutonniere deformity of the PIP joints. The burnt hand will adopt a dysfunctional posture if it is not properly assessed and managed.

- Following the application of grafts, joints may need to be immobilised to allow healing. The therapist should commence assessment when grafts are stable.

## Assessment of scar formation

- The normal healing process involves contracture and scarring. As scarring forms the following problems may develop:
- Reduced ROM due to contraction or adherence to other tissues
- Hard immobile scarring, with possibly raised, hypertrophic areas
- Tight scarring which is uncomfortable, itchy or hypersensitive.

## Psychological status of the patient

- It is important to obtain a good social history and impression of a patient's psychological status.

- Knowledge of pre-injury hobbies, employment and family support systems enables the therapist to set individual goals and treatment plans to maximise a patient's response and compliance.

## Stages of assessment

- In the early stages assessments are carried out in the hospital setting.

- As the patient recovers they may be continued in the outpatient department or in the patient's home environment.

- The later stages of assessment may include consideration of independent function in the home or at work and any adaptations that need to be made.

## Plastic surgery

### Background

- Derived from the Greek *plastikos* which means to mould or to form, defined as:

    *... repairing people and restoring function. It is performed to repair and reshape bodily structures affected by birth defects, developmental abnormalities, trauma/ injuries, infections, tumours and disease (BAPRAS, 2010).*

- Plastic surgery is not just related to cosmetic procedures, e.g. 'tummy tucks' or 'nose jobs'. These procedures comprise about 5% of the total of work done on the NHS, with the majority being reconstructive plastic surgery.

- Plastic surgery may be encountered in many clinical areas:
- Head and neck surgery – ENT
- Craniofacial surgery
- Cleft lip and palate surgery
- Breast surgery
- Trauma
- Oncology
- Orthopaedics
- Hand and upper limb surgery, including brachial plexus and nerve reconstruction.
- The conditions and types of surgery covered in this book are those which would be seen on a typical plastics ward/specialist surgery ward.

## Tendon and nerve injuries

- Patients with tendon injuries tend to be seen by therapists following exploration and reconstructive surgery of any injured structures.
- Although protocols vary depending on the specific unit, patients would tend to come to therapy between 1 and 5 days post surgery. Most units follow an early active movement regime.

## Assessment

### Operation and medical notes

- These will provide information about the social history, past medical history (PMH), medication history (DH) and importantly how the injury occurred.
- These will tell you what structures were repaired, and how they were repaired.
- They will inform you about the state of the structures and whether the repair was deemed to be a strong repair, or if the surgeon requires the repair to be treated with care.
- There may be information relating to any associated injuries. e.g. fractures, or skin loss.

### Talk to the surgeon

- They may be able to provide more information about the patient and the surgery than was recorded on the operation note.

### Revise anatomical knowledge

- It helps to confirm how to test the tendons involved. Have a good textbook available for reference e.g. Muscles, Testing and Function (Kendall and McCreary 1983).
- Know neural anatomy and areas supplied to test nerve function following injury and repair.

### In the assessment area

- The patient may have a bulky bandage and plaster of paris (POP) slab in situ. Flexor tendon repairs will have a POP slab over the dorsum of the arm and fingers, called a 'flexor hood' or 'dorsal slab'.
- Extensor tendon repairs will have a slab on the volar aspect.

- Nerve injuries should be in a volar slab or the arm supported to restrict movement at the repair site.
- In each case, the hand should be in a position of safe immobilisation (POSI) to maintain length in the ligaments.
- The inter phalangeal joints (IPJ) are maintained in neutral extension, the metacarpophalangeal joints (MCPJ) in 50–90° flexion and the thumb in mid-position.
- If the patient does not have a bulky dressing in situ and it states on the operation note that they were put in one after surgery, it is imperative that the tendons are checked to ensure that they are intact.
- Assessment is carried out following a SOAP format (Table 4.2).

## Once the subjective assessment is completed

- Explain what you are about to do
- The last time the patient saw their limb, e.g. hand, it may have been in a traumatic situation. Tell them that you are going to remove their bandage to look at their wounds. They don't have to look, however encourage them to do so, as what they are thinking or imagining is always worse than how their hand actually is.
- Check whether they have eaten before they came to the appointment, and that they don't usually faint when they see wounds. If any doubt exists lie the patient down before removing the dressing.
- Be prepared, it is not good for the patient to hear a sharp intake of breath or a surprised comment when their dressing is removed. This tends to make them more anxious.
- Therapists encounter these wounds on a regular basis; however, 90% of patients have not. If the therapist shows that they are comfortable looking at the wounds, then the patient will feel less anxious. This is one reason for reading the operation notes before the patient's appointment.

### Removing dressings

- Use a sterile environment. Ensure the repaired area (and distal to it) is supported to prevent gravity pulling on the repairs. This is a good habit for the patient to adopt.
- Cut through the bandages on the side away from the wounds and peel back the dressings as this helps to reduce the spread of infection. If the dressing is stuck to the wound it may need soaking off with sterile water.
- Check the wound, is it:
- Surrounded by red areas
- Smelly
- Healing as expected
- White and macerated (a macerated wound is one which has got damp or sweaty and has become waterlogged)
- Clean or dirty
- Oozing or dry (palm wounds can be left open to allow for some ooze to escape)
- In the expected place for the described operation?
- Record everything that is seen, including normal observations and those which will become objective markers. It makes it easier to recall the wound from

**Table 4.2** Subjective Objective Assessment Plan (SOAP) questions and reasoning

| Questions | Why you want to know |
|-----------|----------------------|
| How did they injure/damage the area? | Were they at work? Will this create problems for returning to work? Is there a claim against work? Was it at home – social difficulties? |
| Time between injury and repair? | Ideally a tendon should be repaired within 72 hours. Longer time frames can affect the outcome (Langley and Hobby 2010) |
| Pain presentation: Pain levels | To ensure compliance and good tendon healing, patients need to be doing early exercises. This becomes more difficult if their pain is not adequately controlled |
| Pain descriptions | Nerve pain – burning, electric shocks, deep aching, fizzing<br>Tissue pain – ache, sore, itchy |
| Paraesthesia or anaesthesia | Pins and needles or numbness? May be due to a nerve that was injured and repaired, or is there paraesthesia for another reason? |
| Is there anyone at home with them? | If a tendon injury, they will be unable to use the injured hand for up to 6 weeks (12 weeks before it is fully strong). Are they likely to take off the splint as soon as they get home to make things easier for themselves? |
| Do they smoke? | Nicotine affects the ability of tendons to heal themselves |
| Occupation? | Are they self-employed? Will they have financial difficulties which might mean they go back to work earlier than recommended? Do they get sick pay? |
| Hand dominance? | Which is the injured hand? They may be more compliant if the injured hand is not the dominant hand |
| Past medical history | Have they injured their limb before?<br>What was damaged? This will give an indication of pre-injury function<br>Do they have diabetes? This can affect healing time<br>Any infections which could affect healing? |
| Drug history: medication they are taking | Useful to know if they are on antibiotics post injury – are they taking them?<br>Other analgesia or medication for co-morbidities |

notes when the patient next attends. The size of wounds should be recorded, especially any open areas.

Check the movement of the affected area

• This can be done by:

– Checking the action of the tendons repaired to ensure they are intact

– Tenodesis effect

- Assessing the distance of the fingertips to the distal palmar crease
- Measuring ROM with a goniometer.
- Reassure the patient at every stage that you will not ask them to do anything which would put the surgery at risk.

**Check the sensation of the affected area**

- Often this is not useful in the early stages, as any damaged nerves may be dying back. Recovery usually starts about four weeks after any repair.
- Sensation can be tested in the following ways:
- Semmes Weinstein Monofilament testing (SWMF)
- Two point discrimination
- Temperature control
- Sharp/blunt
- Light touch
- Vibration
- Tinel's test.

## Ongoing assessment

- Following the initial assessment issues for ongoing consideration are:
- Wound healing
- ROM
- Patterns of movement and compensatory movements
- Changes in symptoms
- Function
- Grip and pinch strength
- Scars
- Oedema.
- The individual patient and surgery will determine which are priorities when it comes to ongoing assessment, e.g. if a nerve has been repaired, then changes in symptoms, i.e. loss of sensation and patterns of movement may be more useful than pure ROM.

## Specific reconstructive surgery and repairs

### Replanted digits

- These can include injuries to bones, skin loss, tendon damage, nerve damage and vessels such as the digital arteries and veins, and the common digital vessels.
- A patient will be in hospital for at least a week, to ensure that the finger is 'viable', i.e. it has a good blood supply both in and out of the finger, preventing necrosis.
- Sometimes patients need multiple operations, so the more mobile they get between anaesthetics, the fewer complications occur.

### Skin grafts and muscle flaps

- For defects that have a vascular base and are small enough, a skin graft of varying thickness can be used to close and cover the wound. Muscle flaps are used to cover a defect which does not have a good vascular base.

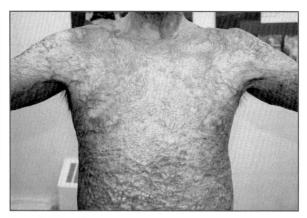

**Figure 4.6** Skin graft.

Skin grafts

- These can be full thickness (down into the dermis) or split thickness (upper layer of skin only).
- The amount of contracture depends on the amount of dermis which is lost. More dermis = more contracture, large defects covered by a skin graft will tend to develop unwanted contractures, affecting later function.
- Skin grafts are taken from areas of the upper thigh, forearm, upper arm or torso. These are called 'donor sites' and heal spontaneously by epithelialisation of the skin cells within 12–14 days.
- Due to the nature of the donor site, these can often be more painful than the graft site as there are exposed nerve endings.
- The skin graft is shaved off the donor area, using either a hand tool or a power dermatome knife. It is then meshed to allow expansion (to cover a larger area) and to allow oedema to escape. It is held in place on the graft site using glue or staples (Figure 4.6).
- The donor site is covered with mefix, which stays in place for 12–14 days.

Muscle flaps

- A muscle flap would be used if there is exposed bone or tendon, or if the defect is too large to be closed with a skin graft.
- The surgeon has to take into account the action that that part of the body has to undergo, e.g. the elbow needs to flex/extend, whilst the back has to undergo much less skin movement. They may cover open tibial fractures, following fracture fixation, or 'fill in a gap' following extensive malignant tissue removal.
- A muscle flap can be free or pedicled, which either means that it is transferred 'free' of its own blood supply, or still fixed to its own blood supply (Table 4.3). If it is a free flap then the flap is anastomosed (fixed) to the blood supply around the affected area. The surgeon needs to ensure that the blood supply at the affected site is adequate, and that the vessels are able to supply the anastomosis.

| Table 4.3 Common muscle flaps | |
|---|---|
| **Type of muscle flap** | **Commonly used for** |
| DIEP (deep inferior epigastric artery) or TRAM (transverse rectus abdominus myocutaneous) flap | Breast reconstruction |
| Gracilis muscle flap | Lower limb trauma and reconstruction with smaller defects |
| Gastrocnemius muscle flap | Lower limb trauma and reconstruction requiring more cover |
| Latissimus dorsi flap | Breast reconstruction Back defects Shoulder or upper arm reconstruction |

- Departments have different systems for managing muscle flaps. This may be a 'dangling' protocol, which involves the patient staying on bed rest with the arm/limb in elevation for 5–7 days.
- During this time the therapist would be expected to:
- Monitor respiratory function
- Provide a bed exercise programme
- Maintain movement in all unaffected joints
- Assess (alongside OTs) the social situation and start making plans for discharge.
- Following a period of bed rest following surgery for a lower limb the patient is encouraged to dangle the leg off the edge of the bed, with the flap being checked to ensure it copes with the influx of blood to the dependent limb. This is begun at 30-second intervals and is increased to 5 minutes over the following 3–5 days.
- Once the patient has passed this point (either with or without dangling), then they will require assessment relating to:
- Mobility
- Social environment and subsequent discharge planning
- Exercises for ROM and strengthening, dependent on the time since surgery and other concurrent injuries
- Oedema management, scar management and continuing mobility dysfunction or compensatory movements.

Breast reconstruction
- Women who have experienced breast cancer and have had a single or double mastectomy may opt to have a reconstruction.
- A reconstruction has been shown to:
- Improve mental health
- Improve emotional well-being
- Improve energy levels
- Give more satisfaction with their appearance following a mastectomy.

**Table 4.4** Advantages of prosthetic and autologous reconstructions

| Prosthetic | Autologous |
|---|---|
| Quick, simple surgery | More natural look |
| Short general anaesthetic and recovery | Most durable reconstruction |
| No operation on healthy tissues | Best cosmetic effect |
| No extra scars | No artificial material used |
| No missing tissue from elsewhere | |

**Table 4.5** Disadvantages of prosthetic and autologous reconstruction

| Prosthetic | Autologous |
|---|---|
| Slow reconstructive process with expansion of implants | Major operation |
| Less symmetry with remaining breast | Extra scars |
| Less natural texture | Complications at the breast and/or donor sites |
| Unsuitable for large breasts | Longer hospital stay |
| Increased risk of infection as artificial materials used | |

- However, there are some who choose not to have a reconstruction due to:
- They feel the flat chest reflects their post-cancer personality better
- They find it difficult to discuss the options, and worry about appearing vain
- They cannot find a surgeon in whom they have confidence
- They find it difficult to cope with more trauma following the diagnosis and treatment for the breast cancer.
- There are two main types of breast reconstruction; a prosthetic implant, or an autologous reconstruction, where skin or tissue from another part of the patient's body is used to reconstruct the breast. There are advantages and disadvantages to each procedure (Tables 4.4 and 4.5), and the choice of surgery is ultimately dependent on patient preference.

## Specific assessment following breast reconstruction

**Post surgery**
- Respiratory check and ongoing maintenance of chest.
- ROM shoulders, back and pelvis, and lower limbs.
- Mobility.
- Core stability once up and mobilising, this is particularly important if the patient has had a TRAM reconstruction.

### Axillary, groin and neck dissections
- Axillary and groin dissections are commonly carried out to remove lymph glands from the area, or to remove adrenal sweat glands for a condition called 'hidradenitis' (excess sweating).

- This can involve extensive surgery around the region, requiring skin grafts or flaps in order to close the remaining tissue.
- Neck dissections are more commonly done for cancer of the mouth, throat or neck itself. They are long operations, and with patients who may be weak as a result of their illness, careful monitoring is required post anaesthetic and following surgery.
- Surgery may involve the use of a radial forearm flap to reconstruct the palate or other parts of the throat or neck, and the hand therapist may be involved in hand and wrist protection in the initial stages which will be progressed to active treatment of the hand and wrist.
- These patients may need a tracheostomy, management of which requires respiratory knowledge and skills. They need to retain an open airway, therefore ability to assess a patient's saturation levels, heart rate (HR), respiratory rate (RR) and knowing the different types of oxygen therapy will assist in the overall assessment of these patients.
- With all dissection patients, the physiotherapist will need to assess:
- ROM of the operated area and the joints above and below
- Pain levels
- Social situation
- Patient's understanding of their condition. Being able to explain to a patient what they have had done requires skill and empathy. The physiotherapist may be the team member that is asked a lot of the questions that the patient did not ask the surgeon. It is important to have a good understanding of surgical procedures and postoperative routines to be able to provide the patient with the answers to any questions they may have.

The references for this chapter can be found on www.expertconsult.com.

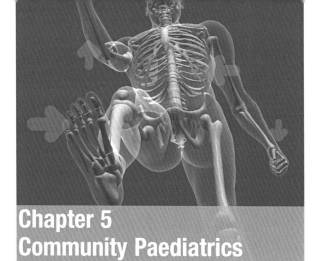

# Chapter 5
# Community Paediatrics

## Introduction

- Community paediatrics involves the assessment of children from neonatal age through to 19 years, with conditions ranging from specific foot problems to complex neurological conditions.

- It is important to have a basic knowledge of child development, milestones and normal movement patterns, knowledge of primitive reflexes and righting reactions.

- The assessment will require the selection of assessment techniques and knowledge that are used in other specialist areas, especially outpatients, orthopaedics, respiratory and neurology.

- To be effective the paediatric physiotherapist has to work with delicately balanced and integrated relationships between children/young people, their parents/carers, educational requirements, medical and therapy needs, personal objectives and anyone else involved in the management of the children.

- These may lead to areas of conflict, which will need to be managed through careful negotiation and all need to be included in planning the development of appropriate goals and functional outcomes, to enable individuals to meet their full potential.

## Venues and appointment times

It is essential to choose a venue to work with children/young people that:
- Has suitable access for wheelchairs, buggies.
- Has a child friendly atmosphere.
- Ensures the safety of both child and therapist.
- Considers travelling distances for families and keeps them to a minimum.

There are a variety of venues a community therapist may work in:

- Child's own home.
- A children's centre, nursery or play group.
- Mainstream school with or without resourced support from the local education authority (LEA).
- Special school.
- Community clinic.
- Some therapists may even consider working in a local gym or other community resources.
- It is also useful to consider the time that an appointment is offered to fit in with family commitments, such as work times for single parents, times other children may need support, e.g. collecting them from school or feeding a baby.

## Consent

- Consent is essential, involving parental consent and also the consent of individuals.
- Therapists often need to consider inventive ways to explain the nature of their assessment and intervention and why it is important, especially to younger children and those with learning difficulties.
- Often a compromise is essential in order to achieve therapy which is effective and efficient, yet compliments the commitment that is made by children and/or those working with them.
- Therapy is often considered to be something that needs to happen 24 hours a day, 7 days a week, being taught and managed by a therapist, but implemented by many others.
- It is especially important to gain parental consent when planning to see a child in school with education staff.
- Children and adolescents often have very strong feelings and may make it clear they do not wish to participate in therapy programmes. It is therefore necessary to try to make treatment sessions fun, but also relevant to meeting set objectives.
- Children should be encouraged to take responsibility for their own therapy if this is possible.
- All health and social care organisations have guidelines or policies on consent. It is essential for any physiotherapist working in this field to familiarise themselves with these from the outset of the time they are working in community paediatric practice.

## Child protection/safeguarding

- Child protection is very high on the agenda of everyone who works in paediatrics.
- Closely linked to nationally driven policies and procedures all health and social care organisations offer essential training to support therapists in this area.
- These are in place not just to protect children, but also to protect those working with them.

- There are many forms of abuse that children can be subjected to and a therapist working with children will often be the first to identify a possible problem.

- It is the responsibility of the individual to ensure that they attend child protection training as a priority to equip themselves with the knowledge to identify and handle these situations correctly.

- It is important to remember initiating a child protection procedure or a Common Assessment Framework (CAF) does not mean that children will be taken away from their families, very often it will flag up that a family needs help and identifies how it can be provided.

- All therapists are in a position of trust, but it is prudent that a physiotherapist does not put themselves into a situation where they are working alone with a child.

- As therapists we often handle children, ensure people know what you are going to do and why and if they find this unacceptable look for another way or even a completely different activity.

## Manual handling and risk assessment

- It is an essential part of therapy practice to ensure the safety of those we work with and ourselves. All trusts have robust policies and procedures to ensure safe practice and it is an individual therapist's responsibility to ensure that they attend patient handling training and relevant updates on a regular basis (CSP 2008).

- A risk assessment will need to be completed for any therapeutic handling procedure to ensure any risk to the health of the therapist or the child is reduced as far as is reasonably practicable.

## Statements of special educational need

- For those children with a physical difficulty, integrating therapy programmes into many education settings can often be tricky.

- If a child has a statement of special educational needs (this is a legally binding document that requires the LEA to provide specific support over and above that provided for most children, in terms of extra finance and consideration of appropriate school placement) to support their passage through school.

- It is essential to ensure that a physiotherapy report is included within this.

- There will be opportunities to outline what a child is able to do and where and what kind of help they will need to develop physical and mobility skills in their school setting.

- If they are going to need postural support equipment in school this is the time to say so, pointing out when and for how long it should be used and who would be expected to pay for and maintain it.

- At this point the physiotherapist will be expected to say how much 'hands on' therapy support the child should expect to receive to meet their full potential.

- It must be pointed out that it may not be possible to provide the desired frequency of therapeutic input.

- Therapy and health issues are usually placed in part 5 of a child's statement and cannot be challenged at an educational tribunal.

- If parents have issues with therapy provision as it stands in a statement they need to take this up with your organisation/trust.
- It must be realised that it is not the personal responsibility of the physiotherapist to provide what is outlined in the statement.

## Physiotherapy in mainstream schools

- For most schools therapy is usually not a primary consideration.
- Often integrating this into a busy school curriculum is a real juggling act and gets harder the further a child progresses through the school system.
- It is surprisingly difficult to convince teachers that if a child has completed their physiotherapy programme they are more prepared and comfortable to apply themselves to learning.
- Another case needs to be made for placing the child in an appropriate piece of postural supporting equipment because this will enable the child to complete tasks more effectively and efficiently.

## Physiotherapy in a school setting

- In a school setting it is relatively easy to integrate therapy into the fun learning situations which are created for younger children.
- Most education staff are happy to do so if you explain to them how and why.
- However with brighter children school staff often feel that time should be spent specifically on learning rather than on time-consuming therapy-related activities, however integrated they may be, especially as they grow older and school targets become more important.
- There are issues associated with placement in a nursery or school. These are wide ranging and will change as a child grows and expectations change.
- It is essential to provide specific training for staff and equipment to enable a child to be able to sit, stand, mobilise and function in a way that is not hazardous to themselves, other children or staff.
- As a child progresses through education there are issues of negotiating a larger building with dispersed classrooms on multiple levels.
- Appendices 5.1, 5.2 and 5.3 cover some of the commonly encountered issues in nurseries and in schools with suggestions for how these can be managed satisfactorily.

## Assessment of the child

- It is helpful to be familiar with specific classification and assessment tools such as;
- Gross Motor Function Measure (GMFM)
- Gross Motor Classification System (GMFCS)
- Movement ABC
- Paediatric Evaluation of Disability Inventory (PEDI)
- Chailey
- Pain assessments
- Assisting hand assessments.
- These are useful once the main problems of the child have been established.

Please see chapter 1 for additional material on motor disorders

# Referral process and preparation for the assessment

- Every community paediatric service will have a 'new referral' procedure and it is important to be familiar with this.
- Always check that the contact details on a referral are correct.
- If speaking to the family on the phone prior to the assessment confirm information such as;
- Child's name and date of birth
- Address
- Contact number
- GP details
- School
- Other professionals involved
- Equipment.
- Explain what the assessment appointment will involve, give the parents your contact details and inform them how to cancel the appointment should it become necessary.
- Arrange a convenient appointment with the family; try not to see the child when it is due a sleep or is hungry as this is likely to affect willingness to cooperate and/or play.
- Before arranging to visit a child's home it is essential to be familiar with the service-specific lone-working policy.
- Before assessing a child access other medical records and/or have a discussion with other professionals involved with the child.
- It is also useful to research any presenting diagnosis in order to be well informed during the assessment.
- On the day of the assessment ring or text to confirm that the child will be attending.
- Parents often find it difficult to remember the age that their child achieved various milestones.
- The 'Personal Child Health Record', often known as the red book, has pages for parents to record their child's development and therefore it is useful if this is available during the assessment.

## Equipment to have at assessment
- Goniometer.
- Tape measure.
- Notepad and pen.
- Assessment forms if used by your service.
- Appropriate toys/activities for the child's age and cognitive ability.
- Gloves and apron and alcohol gel should be available.

## Environment
- When planning an assessment consider the best environment for the assessment to take place.
- The environments available to you will largely depend on where in the community the child is assessed, e.g. school (SFN/mainstream), home, health centre.

- Wherever the assessment takes place it is important that the environment is warm and safe.
- Privacy is important as the child/young person may have to be undressed or the parents/caregivers may disclose confidential information.
- Consider Health and Safety; is a hoist required, would a therapy couch or mat be most suitable, will space be required to observe walking, running, jumping?
- Is the child likely to put things in its mouth?

## Subjective assessment

### Background information

- Obtaining a comprehensive history of the child's condition and progress to date will 'help' you to decide how to proceed with your assessment.
- Some of the information required can often be obtained from previous records.
- Discussion with the parents/caregivers and child, if they have the cognitive ability, will provide an insight into the child's general health, well-being and life skills.
- It will also establish expectations of the child, parents and school.
- Some questions may be upsetting for a family, especially if the assessment is before they have been given a reason for their child's difficulties or if they are anxious about their child.
- It is important that the family/carers and child understand the questions; therefore they should be concise and relevant, avoiding jargon.
- An interpreter is recommended if either parent is not fluent in English.
- Before the assessment it is good practice to explain what will happen during the assessment and consent must be obtained before proceeding.
- Consent must be documented appropriately in accordance with local policies.

### Questions

- What are the parents' main concerns?
- When did they first have concerns?

### Birth history

- Any complications during pregnancy?
- Scan results.
- Labour; type, duration, complications.
- Apgar score at birth.
- Was baby given to mum immediately post delivery?
- Was baby with mum on ward?
- Discharge timing.

### Developmental history

- Missing a developmental stage can influence a child's gross motor abilities, e.g. a child who does not crawl may have poor proximal stability.
- Achievement of milestones – smiling, rolling, sitting, crawling, pull to stand, walk.
- Has there been any regression in their abilities?
- Did the baby have time on its stomach?

- Did the child crawl?
- Did the child use a baby walker?
- Any difficulties with feeding?
- Any history of respiratory problems?

Medical history
- Diagnosis (if known)
- General health
- Other medical conditions such as epilepsy, asthma, reflux
- Surgery
- Investigations and results (if known) – including scans and X-rays
- Medications
- Orthotics
- Other professionals involved.

Family history
- Siblings? What ages, are they healthy?
- Incidence of similar conditions/difficulties within the extended family.
- Consanguinity.

Education
- Name of school/nursery attended – contact details of SENCO and LSA.
- Do they have an Educational Statement?
- Equipment used at school (including manual handling).
- How they manage in PE, lunchtime and playtime?
- Ease of accessing the school including how they manage between classes.
- Any specific difficulties.

Social
- Hobbies.
- Likes/dislikes.

ADL activities
- What do they find difficult?
- What would they like to be able to do?
- How much help does the child need during activities such as;
- Mobility
- Dressing/ undressing
- Toileting
- Eating.
- How well do they sleep?
- Do they use a sleep system?
- Are they in pain? – if so – where, how often, intensity what helps?

## Objective assessment

- Observational analysis of a child's movement should occur whilst they enter the assessment area, in the assessment environment and during play.

- Observe:
- Head, trunk, and limb posture
- Eye contact
- Movement patterns
- Voluntary and involuntary movements
- Influence of retained primitive reflexes
- Symmetry
- Balance
- Ability to weight bear through upper limbs
- Transitions, e.g. movement from lying to sitting
- Fluidity of movement
- Muscle hypertrophy or atrophy
- Use of hands during activities and play:
a Communication skills
b Behaviour
c Relationship with parents and/or caregivers, and siblings present at the assessment.
- Observation gives the child time to adjust to the environment and enables a rapport to be developed between the therapist and child.
- Discover what type of activities or toys they like, before starting the assessment.

## Physical assessment

- Ideally the child should be undressed; however, this may not always be possible, e.g. lack of privacy.
- Taking a young child from a parent's lap may upset the child significantly and curtail any physical assessment.
- It is possible to assess much of the child on the mother's lap and slowly persuade the child to partake in other activities.
- The activities chosen will depend on the child's age and ability.
- Analyse the quality of the function, not just the ability to succeed.
- The starting point of the assessment will depend on the child's ability and willingness to be 'handled'.

### Supine

- Observe posture recording asymmetries.
- Record abnormal movements/posture, e.g. flexion, adduction and internal/ external rotation of hips, thumb in palms, fisted hands.
- General feel of all limbs for joint range and muscle tone.
- Note any resistance and consider cause.
- Is the end feel normal, bony or due to soft tissue limitation?
- Is the direction of the movement normal?
- Measure active ROM using a goniometer and muscle strength using Oxford scale noting abnormality or asymmetry.
- If a child presents with increased tone, check for the dynamic ranges of muscles.

- Note any clonus.
- Check leg length.

## Prone
- Observe posture, movement and asymmetries in prone.
- Prone is the best position to measure hip rotation, as it is easier to control movement at the pelvis.

## Side lying
- For the child more severely affected by a neuromuscular condition assess whether the child can be placed in this position.
- Note if they are able to bring their hands to midline, together, and to their mouth.
- Does the child use side lying during their transitional movements?

## Sitting
- Assess floor sitting as well as sitting on a stool/chair.
- Does the child have to be placed in these positions or can they achieve them independently?
- How much support does the child need to maintain the position, and where is the support required?
- Analyse posture and movement as for the previous positions.
- How good is head control?
- Does the child use fixation strategies to maintain the position?
- Is there a scoliosis or kyphosis and is it postural or fixed?
- How good is their balance, e.g. can they reach out of their base of support?
- Are they able to move in and out of sitting?

### Assess and analyse other general gross motor activities as appropriate
- Floor mobility.
- Rolling.
- Crawling.
- Standing – check spinal posture.
- Sit to stand.
- Floor to stand – Check for Gower's sign.
- Walking – with and without orthoses.
- Transitions.
- Standing on one leg.
- Stairs.
- Running.
- Jumping.
- Hopping.
- Skipping.
- Kicking.
- Catching.

- Hand function; e.g. grasp, co-ordination, movement of wrist and fingers, writing.

## Video recording

- Video recording can be useful to aid analysis of movement patterns, remember written consent must be gained from the parents first.

## Sensory assessment

- The brain integrates information about sights, sounds, textures, smells, tastes and movements that are perceived in an organised way to assign meaning to sensory experiences and formulates response and behaviour accordingly.
- In the normally developing child sensory integration occurs when the child participates in everyday activities, with a child's love for sensory activities fuelling an inner drive and motivation to conquer challenges (Murray-Slutsky and Paris, 2005). A child explores the environment, tries new activities and strives to meet increasingly more complex challenges.
- Mastering new challenges gives a child the confidence to try more difficult tasks.
- Different responses:
- Over responsive (hyper-responsive), a child registers sensation too intensely.
- Under responsive (hyporesponsive), a child's sensory system is not responsive to information in their environment.
- The senses/sensory system:
- Touch – tactile system
- Sight – vision
- Hearing – auditory system
- Smell
- Taste.
- Additional senses include proprioception and movement (vestibular).

## Treatment planning

- On completion of the assessment it should be possible to identify a list of problems on which the treatment plan can be based.
- These may not be motor problems, e.g. they may be poor communication or severe epilepsy
- These need to be documented as they may affect the treatment plan and also it is important that other members of staff are made aware of them.
- It is important to discuss findings with the child's parents/carers so that they can clarify issues and gain a better understanding of the problems.
- Joint goal setting is very important as it gives the child and family ownership of the objectives; it also allows the child, family and physiotherapist to understand their personal commitments to the treatment plan.
- Identify whether the child needs referral to any other services and discuss this with the family.
- Assessment findings should be recorded in accordance with organisational and professional body requirements.

- A copy of the assessment should be sent to the parents and their consent gained for this to be distributed to other professionals.

## Respiratory

- Children may have respiratory problems for a variety of reasons; some directly related to their condition, others as a separate issue.
- These could impact on their growth, development and health and will need addressing as part of the whole assessment.
- It is important to recognise respiratory dysfunction to provide early intervention and hopefully prevent admission to hospital.
- The primary purpose of a respiratory assessment is to determine the adequacy of gas exchange, which is oxygenation of the tissues and excretion of carbon dioxide.
- By undertaking a respiratory assessment in the community physiotherapists are in the position to act on findings and ensure that appropriate medical and/or physiotherapy interventions are initiated.
- The severity of the respiratory condition can vary greatly from having little or no impact on daily life to having a significant impact, which can lead to modification of individual treatment plans.
- It is important to understand the state of the condition, i.e. is it controlled and/or stable to uncontrolled and/or deteriorating.
- All respiratory conditions are monitored through GPs, or paediatricians, or respiratory consultants therefore good communication is necessary to be appropriately informed about any treatment decisions made by health professionals and parents, particularly with regard to resuscitation plans.

## Ask, look, listen, feel, smell

### Ask

- History:
- Hospital admissions due to chest (how many?)
- Family history of respiratory problems (e.g. asthma)
- Recurrent chest infections
- Breathing difficulties
- Failure to thrive
- Poor feeding (breathless or sweaty whilst feeding)
- Poor swallow
- Reflux
- Aspiration problems
- Exercise tolerance
- Cyanosis
- Episodes of apnoea
- Wheeze/cough
- ENT symptoms
- Drugs
- Mentation – child's state, i.e. anxious
- Previous chest X-ray

- Any other professionals involved for any of the above?
- Any equipment used for chest? Ventilator (night and/or daytime), Suction (when and how often is it used?). Nebulisers.
• Be aware of any agreed resuscitation plans for individual children.

Look
• General observation:
- Well/unwell
- Awake/alert
- Increased drowsiness can lead to unconsciousness.
- Distressed generally
- Temperature (normal or raised)
- Effort/work of breathing
- Signs of respiratory distress. Children who have neuromuscular disease may present in respiratory failure without increased effort of breathing.
- Chest deformity
- Positioning
- Rashes.
• Hands:
- Clubbing of finger nails
- Colour of finger nails
- Tremor
- Capillary refill
- Radial pulse if possible
- Nutritional state.
• Face:
- Colour, generally of face
- Lip colour.
• Nose:
- Blocked up nose
- Snotty/red
- Flaring nostrils
- Abdomen (pushing out as child breathes out).
• Neck:
- Lymph nodes
- Trachea, is it central?
• Chest:
- Ribs (looking more prominent as child breathes)
- Recession, subcostal/intercostal
- Harrison's sulcus – two symmetrical sulci, horizontal, at the lower margin of the anterior thorax, at the attachment of the diaphragm. A sign of prolonged respiratory distress in children. Most commonly present in children with asthma who have required an increased respiratory effort over several months.
- Accessory muscle use

- Oximetry if available
- Gasping, call 999.

Listen
- Audible noise:
- Sounds from the child/chest audible to ear is upper respiratory tract
- Crackles (Rice Krispies)
- Wheeze (whistling noise breathing out)
- Grunting
- Stridor (whistling noise breathing in).
- Auscultation if possible:
- Appropriate-size stethoscope needed
- Size and age of child
- Musculoskeletal deformity
- Breath sounds
- Added sounds
- Asymmetrical sounds
- Pleural rub (squeaky).
- Cough:
- Effective?
- Productive?
- Dry?
- Fruity?

Feel (with hands)
- Chest movement:
- Symmetrical movement
- Inspiration
- Expiration
- Respiratory rate
- Pulse/heart rate
- Fremitus/crepitus = secretions.

Smell
- Odours:
- Breath odours.

## Signs of respiratory distress

- Breathing rate, rapid and shallow and an increase in the number of breaths per minute may indicate that a person is having trouble breathing or not getting enough oxygen.
- Heart rate, tachycardia (fast heart rate).
- Colour changes, a bluish colour seen around the mouth, on the inside of the lips, or on the fingernails may occur when a person is not getting as much oxygen as needed.

- The colour of the skin may also appear pale or grey.
- Grunting can be heard each time the person exhales.
- This grunting is the body's way of trying to keep air in the lungs so they will remain inflated, needs urgent attention.
- Nose flaring while breathing may indicate that a person is having to work harder to breathe.
- Retractions, the chest appears to sink in just below the neck and/or under the sternum with each breath – as the child tries to bring more air into their lungs.
- Sweating, may be increased on the head, but the skin does not feel warm to the touch.
- More often, the skin may feel cool or clammy, especially when the breathing rate is fast.
- Wheezing, a whistling or musical sound heard with each breath may indicate that the air passages may be constricted, making it more difficult to breathe.
- Irritability, there may be a change in mental state due to hypoxaemia, which leads to irritability in children.

## Cardiorespiratory values

- Oxygen saturation 90–98% = normal range.
- Respiratory rates (breaths per minute) (Table 5.1).
- Heart rates (awake) (Table 5.2).
- Systolic blood pressure (mmHg) (Table 5.3).
- It is essential to know normal values of heart rate, respiratory rate ($O_2$ % if available) and patterns of breathing for the more severely affected children especially if a change of position has an impact on breathing.
- This status should be regularly monitored for change and/or deterioration (parents, carers and learning support assistants can be trained to recognise changes).

**Table 5.1** Paediatric respiratory rates (breaths per minute) (ALSG 2005)

| | |
|---|---|
| Neonate | 40–60 |
| Less than 1 year | 30–40 |
| 1–5 years | 25–35 |
| 5–12 years | 20–25 |
| Older than 12 years | 15–20 |

**Table 5.2** Paediatric heart rates (beats per minute) (ALSG 2005)

| | |
|---|---|
| Neonate | 100–200 |
| Less than 1 year | 110–160 |
| 1–2 years | 100–150 |
| 2–5 years | 95–140 |
| 5–12 years | 80–120 |
| Older than 12 years | 60–100 |

**Table 5.3** Paediatric blood pressure values (mmHg) (ALSG 2005)

| | |
|---|---|
| Neonate | 60–90 |
| Less than 1 year | 70–90 |
| 1–2 years | 80–95 |
| 2–5 years | 80–100 |
| 5–12 years | 90–110 |
| Older than 12 years | 100–120 |

- Documenting values can provide evidence of patterns, changes and deterioration that can result in referral to paediatric clinic or justification for the purchase of equipment for managing respiratory conditions.
- Children are a diverse group of people. They vary enormously in weight, size, shape, intellectual ability and emotional response.
- Children are different to adults in the following areas:
- Weight
- Anatomical – size and shape
- Physiological – cardiovascular, respiratory, immune function
- Psychological – intellectual ability, emotional response.

**It is important to note**

- Absolute size and relative body proportions change with age.
- Observations of children must be related to their age.
- Therapy in children must be related to their age and weight.
- Special psychological needs of children must be considered.

## Cardiac/respiratory arrest

- Cardiac arrest in children is rarely due to primary cardiac disease.
- This differs from adults where the primary arrest is often cardiac and circulatory and respiratory function may remain near normal until the moment of arrest.
- In children most cardiorespiratory arrests are secondary to hypoxia caused by:
- Respiratory pathology
- Birth asphyxia
- Inhalation of a foreign body
- Bronchiolitis
- Asthma.
- Respiratory arrest also occurs secondary to neurological dysfunction caused by events such as:
- Convulsions
- Poisoning
- Raised intracranial pressure (ICP), e.g. head injury or acute encephalopathy.

- Symptoms of nocturnal failure:
- Daytime sleepiness
  Behaviour changes
- Morning headaches
- Fatigue
- Difficulty sleeping
- Needing frequent re-positioning overnight.

## Respiratory rate (RR)

- Increased respiratory rate indicates possible airway disease.
- Slowing or slow RR indicates breathing fatigue.

## Recession

- As children have a more compliant chest wall (not as rigid as adults) any ↑ negative pressure in thorax will result in intercostal, subcostal or sternal recession.
- Greater recession = greater respiratory distress.

## Stridor

- More pronounced on inspiration, but may occur during expiration.
- Indicates upper airway obstruction.
- Always consider possible foreign body inhalation.

## Wheeze

- Wheeze may subside with exhaustion.

## Grunting

- A grunting child indicates an attempt to keep the distal airways open by generating a grunt, i.e. positive end expiratory pressure.
- It is also a sign of increasing respiratory distress.

## Accessory muscles

- A child may use the sternomastoid muscles to assist breathing.
- In infants this may lead to bobbing of their head.

## Oximetry

- 95–100% on room air.
- Is this normal for the child?

## Heart rate

- Bradycardia:
- Defined as a heart rate (HR) below 60 or a rapidly falling HR with poor systemic perfusion.
- Consider when to start cardiac compressions on a falling HR, i.e. below 50 with signs of poor perfusion.
- Tachycardia:
- A heart rate that exceeds the normal range for a resting heart rate, due to; hypoxia, anxiety or fever.

### Colour

- Hypoxia
  - Leads to peripheral vasoconstriction and eventually cyanosis
  - Once the cyanosis is evident centrally (think smurf) the child is close to respiratory arrest.

### Mentation

- As a child's respiratory distress evolves they become anxious.
- Increased drowsiness and fatigue grows.
- Ask parents if this is normal.
- If parents are concerned then you should be.

The references for this chapter can be found on www.expertconsult.com.

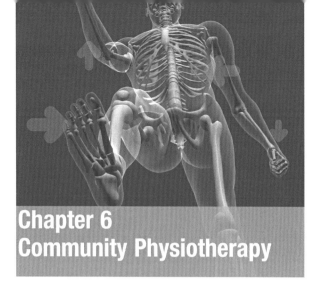

# Chapter 6
# Community Physiotherapy

## Introduction

- Community physiotherapy can be offered to people who are likely to benefit most from treatment in their own environment.

- Those who are housebound or have a long-term condition are examples of where this may be more appropriate than seeing them in a formal setting.

- A community physiotherapist can work in many different capacities, as a single-handed domiciliary physiotherapist, part of a multidisciplinary multiagency intermediate care team (ICT) or in one of the many other community teams.

- The assessment can take place in a variety of settings, from privately owned housing, rented accommodation, Council or Housing Association accommodation, supported housing (sheltered or special sheltered), a caravan, hostel, residential/nursing home or a day centre.

- Careful consideration must be given to the patient's choice (DOH 2001a), culture (CRE 2002), privacy, dignity and confidentiality (DOH 2003) (this includes never leaving messages on an answer-phone without the patient's permission).

- To ensure a safe interaction for the patient and physiotherapist a risk assessment needs to be carried out to cover the physiotherapist entering a person's home environment alone, with the difficulties this brings in terms of the potential for providing treatment in the space available (CSP 1998, 2002, 2009a,b).

- The environmental constraints where treatments take place could include the room being confined by furniture and general clutter such as piles of old newspapers or magazines. The room may be generally unkempt or even unclean and may be completely unsuitable for hospital equipment that requires space and a smooth clear floor to operate safely.

- Community physiotherapy is a speciality which requires 'core' physiotherapy assessment and treatment skills, with the additional focus on home-based functional goals.

- The functional goals are related to the patient's specific needs and their environment. If appropriate this can involve family members or carers to ensure that as much information as possible is obtained in order that the intervention will provide maximum benefit for the patient.

- Some physiotherapists find adjusting to this non-traditional approach frustrating or difficult, as there can be a considerable reduction in the time that they are able to use their 'pure' physiotherapy skills. The different working practice involves the development of new skills in holistic assessment, a more functional approach to treatment, the ability to set goals with the patient, that may be biased towards the patient's needs rather than the desired physiotherapy outcomes. The role may even involve the physiotherapist being an advocate for the patient.

- Where consent is required for involvement with carers, either formal (through an agency) or informal (family or friends) this must be clarified as part of the assessment process (CSP 2004, DOH, 2001b,c,d).

- When visiting the patient in their home environment the physiotherapist may encounter issues around the patient being a vulnerable adult and these issues need to be identified and addressed appropriately (DOH, 2001a). Potential protection of vulnerable adults and safeguarding issues need to be identified and addressed appropriately (DOH 2006, ISA 2010). There are many types of abuse that may be encountered in the community setting, for example; neglect, physical, emotional, psychological and financial abuse (DCA 2005).

- A thorough assessment may need to take place over several visits; this will depend on the patient's ability to engage in the process. The limitations could be due to concentration span, exercise tolerance, mental state or other factors.

- Some community therapy teams may only be able to offer a brief intervention, consisting of assessment and advice. This will involve the physiotherapist undertaking a more specific, but superficial assessment to determine a patient's problems.

- If more complex issues are identified and a comprehensive assessment is required, this may need to be discussed within the team resulting in a request for a further referral or intervention by another team with a particular expertise.

- It is helpful for the physiotherapist to have an understanding of how teams in the community may differ in their roles. Social services teams will need to follow their directive regarding the types of issues they can deal with. If a patient has substantive needs then this becomes a priority for the service. Decisions need to be made about the referral of a patient with moderate needs and whether they will be able to access the service.

- It is important to be aware of other services that are available in the local area, statutory, voluntary organisations, charities and self-help groups (Appendix 6.1).

## Referrals

- Depending on the criteria for each particular service, the referral could originate from any of the following: primary, secondary or tertiary care, social services, the voluntary sector or in some instances self-referral. With this in mind it is essential that the reason for referral is clear, realistic and has been agreed with the patient.

- In addition to the required standard data the referral form should include information about the social history of the patient, access to the property and any known risks to staff.

- To supplement the referral information the GP can supply other medical records (hard copy or electronic), which can include medical history, details of next of kin, name of preferred contact, current medication as well as any previous interventions or other referrals.

- For patients referred following an acute episode of care in hospital, for example, following surgery or a fracture fixation, it is essential to confirm relevant dates for fracture healing times, or precautions following joint replacement surgery.

## Knowledge for the community

### Patient choice

- Many patients choose to request physiotherapy, but referrals made solely to satisfy the patient (or their carers), when the proposed goals are not realistic, can be frustrating for both sides. On occasions a referral can give the patient a false expectation of the potential benefits that can be gained from physiotherapy intervention.

- Some patients will have been seen previously by other services, including community physiotherapy and it is important to be aware of previous treatment approaches and the outcome of these as it may be possible to use the information as a basis for deciding the best intervention for the patient's current episode.

- Some patients may chose not to engage with the intervention and this must be respected, documented and reported back to the referrer.

- If, on assessment, it becomes apparent that the patient is not willing to continue with the proposed intervention, e.g. home exercise programme, then this decision must be explored further with the patient and the potential issues that may arise must be clearly outlined to them. The content of the discussion and the agreed outcomes must be documented.

### Culture

- Develop an awareness of cultural requirements of patients to ensure the treatment is appropriate to their lifestyle.

- The choice of the individual to carry out a task in a specific way that might not be in accordance with the therapy plan must be acknowledged.

- Do not make assumptions, ask the patient about their preference for treatment that is appropriate to their culture and lifestyle. For example, if there is need to wash under running water it is inappropriate to set the goal for strip-washing at a basin. If it is not culturally acceptable to access the kitchen, then this needs to be taken into account when planning treatment interventions.

### Confidentiality

- It is not appropriate to leave a message on an answerphone when attempting to make a first appointment to visit a patient.

- During the assessment confirm with the patient that it is acceptable or practical to leave messages on an answerphone or mobile phone. In addition clarify if a third party is involved in listening to messages, such as a family member, neighbour or warden.

- Privacy must be respected. As a community physiotherapist you will be working as a guest in someone's home and as such you must respect their wish for privacy and lifestyle choices.

- It is necessary to explain to the patient what the assessment process will involve and if the patient wishes to have others present, either their family or friend or another member of staff during the consultation then this wish must be respected.

- Just as you would close curtains around a patient's bed on the ward or in the department for privacy, remember bedrooms and living rooms may be overlooked by other houses or even be on a bus route, where passengers may be able to see into the accommodation.

- Respect a patient's dignity at all times. A patient may feel more relaxed in their own surroundings, but may need more time to complete tasks. A physiotherapist should be conscious of not rushing a patient, to maintain the dignity of the patient an assessment may need to be spread over several sessions.

- Others present during assessment and subsequent treatment should only be there with the consent of the patient.

## Risk assessment

- It is essential that there are effective risk management procedures in place to ensure that personal safety, lone working, moving and handling, environmental and other risks are assessed and appropriate action plans identified.

- Therapists should ensure that they are familiar with and adhere to local policies and procedures (CSP 1998, 2002, 2009a,b).

### Lone working and personal safety

- Often staff will be working alone for at least part of the day.

- If there are electronic community records it is important that these are accessed to establish if there are any noted concerns regarding the patient before the initial visit.

- If possible, telephone the patient prior to visiting to confirm the address, any parking restrictions, access to the property and whether the patient will be alone or have family or friends present.

### Moving and handling

- Statutory training provided annually by employers or universities covers the basic legal requirements for you to ensure your safety and that of the patient.

- Equipment is available and must be used if indicated as a result of the risk assessment.

- Techniques used by the family and/or patient must be reviewed and if unsafe or inappropriate techniques are being used these must be addressed and safer alternatives agreed and documented. If agreement cannot be reached with the patient and/or carers, then it is essential to record this.

- A physiotherapist must never put themselves at risk of injury or harm.

## Environment

- Points to consider:
- Is the property in a high-risk area?
- Is there safe parking nearby?
- Is there safe access to the property (communal entrances/uneven paths)?
- Is the property self-contained or communal living (hostel or B&B)?
- Is there an entry phone, key-safe or on-site warden?
- Is the patient safe to open the door independently or does the patient live alone or with family?
- Are there pets or vermin, that could pose a risk?
- Is there adequate heating, lighting and ventilation?
- Is the environment cluttered or dirty?
- Are there continence issues, which could result in a wet floor or bed?
- Are there trip hazards, rugs/mats/loose flooring/cables?
- Are there any moving and handling risks, e.g. the height of bed, chair/ toilet?
- Is the environment suitable for equipment, if necessary?
- How is equipment delivered in your area?

## Important safety considerations

- Always check the reliability of information as far as possible.
- Do not visit a patient alone if you have any underlying anxiety or concern.
- End an intervention immediately, if you feel threatened.
- Have a planned exit strategy ready should you need it.
- It is not recommended to assess a new patient at the end of the working day. It is advisable to do these new assessments during the working day when colleagues are aware of your whereabouts and the unknown environment and patient can be managed with minimal risk.
- Ensure parking area is well lit and avoid isolated underground parking whenever possible (Figure 6.1).

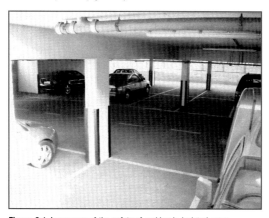

**Figure 6.1** Awareness of the safety of parking in isolated areas.

## Assessment process

- In many communities the single assessment process is used as a joint Health and Social Services assessment tool, which can be supplemented with multidisciplinary and specialist physiotherapy assessments.

- When the assessment is complete it will be a 'snap-shot' in time and it is essential in community work to contextualise this information.

- Focus on the reason for referral, including any long-term issues and functional limitations and how these are currently being managed is essential before identifying how the new issues can be addressed.

### Consent

- Consent to share any information must be obtained from the patient at assessment. Patient-held notes in the community are a useful resource, but the wishes of the patient as to whom has access to these must be respected (CSP 2004, DOH, 2001b,c,d).

- Communication will be more difficult with patients who do not have English as a first language. Translation services should be available, but it may not be possible to access this service for some dialects. Local policies recommend that family members or friends are not used and that trained translators should be used for confidentiality, accuracy and maintenance of the patient's dignity.

- Contact details and written information/advice should be left with the patient in a place agreed by them to ensure confidentiality.

- Patients with any communication problems, e.g. sensory impairment, low literacy skills or other challenges need to be managed in an appropriate way.

- Once communication channels and previous interventions have been established, relevant subjective information for the intervention needs to be gathered.

## Subjective assessment

- As with any physiotherapy intervention, consent is legally required prior to each part of the assessment and subsequent sharing of information.

- Most physiotherapy assessments carried out in the community follow the biopsychosocial model.

### Medical history

- Demographic information, past and current medical history as well as medication information is readily available and will have been recorded in the records of the patient held by Health and Social Services.

- Community physiotherapists have the opportunity and responsibility to obtain the maximum amount of relevant information to influence assessment, goal setting and subsequent treatment.

- Time restrictions may have prevented previous professionals from gaining 'in-depth' and sometimes personal information, which may impact on the management of the patient.

- The community physiotherapist should be able to give the patient the time to focus on and explore aspects of their physical and mental well-being to enable an effective assessment to be completed.

- Effective assessment helps to establish an effective treatment plan and therefore leads to improvements in the quality of life of the patient.

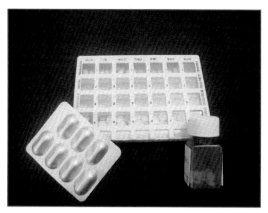

**Figure 6.2** Compliance aids, Dossette box.

## Drug history

- All patients should have a regular medication review, during the assessment check that the patient is taking their medication according to the instructions and report any deviation from the plan to the GP.
- Polypharmacy can be confusing, so compliance aids, e.g. blister packs or the use of a dossette box may be appropriate if it has been identified that the medication regimen is not being managed safely (Figure 6.2).
- It is essential to check that patients can access their medication, either from conventional bottles or the compliance aid.
- Check local policies to see if formal carers are trained to administer medication from specific containers (bottles or compliance aids).

## Pain

- Using core assessment skills will reveal if pain is impacting on functional activities of daily living.
- Management of pain is closely linked with the medication regimen, so consider the 24-hour pain cycle. Having the morning dose of analgesia by the bedside ready for the morning can impact greatly on a patient's ability to undertake the first tasks of the day.
- As with other medication it is important that these are taken regularly and the maximum dose is not exceeded in any 24-hour period.

## Range of movement and muscle strength

- Core assessment skills will be used, but may need to be adapted for use in the community setting. Often working with a client group with long-term conditions and/or chronic reduced levels of function make it difficult to improve functional ability with an exercise programme.

- Having the time to discuss the impact of these limitations and restrictions on their preferred activity level should guide, inform and influence goal setting, e.g. patients in single-level living accommodation will still need to do steps in order to access amenities in other locations.

- If the patient agrees there may need to be simple environmental adaptations, such as adapting the height of a chair, bed or toilet seat and ensuring items in the kitchen are within reach.

- Remember that there is now increasing availability of simple equipment in high street stores. If a referral onto statutory services is not appropriate or wanted by the patient, then advice regarding suitability of privately purchased equipment can be given after the assessment has been completed.

## Decreased exercise tolerance (respiratory or cardiac impairment)

- Patients may describe feeling frail and having less energy.

- This gradual deconditioning may be improved with a progressive exercise programme.

- If this is not appropriate, or the patient does not choose to participate, referral to Occupational Therapy should be considered for energy conservation techniques or provision of equipment, e.g. placing a stool or chair in the bathroom or kitchen which may facilitate independence.

## Mobility

- Patients should be given time to express concerns about the impact of any decrease in their mobility that has affected their lifestyle.

- Assessment needs to identify if the patient is safe to access all areas of their home environment or if there needs to be an alteration to single-level living or even the setting up of a microenvironment (where the patient is able to access all facilities in one room).

- Previous equipment provision and advice needs to be reviewed. There may be a change in the patient's condition and therefore the previously supplied walking aids may need to be replaced.

- Patients with less than substantial needs may need to be advised to purchase mobility aids privately.

- After an acute event, e.g. fall or fracture, timely and specific assessment is essential for reducing the risk of further falls and increasing confidence in mobility and improving their quality of life and psychological state (DOH, 2001a).

- When gathering information on their falls history, the community physiotherapist will be in the ideal situation to assess the home environment for potential hazards.

- High-level function related to outdoor mobility and the use of public and private transport can be considered for inclusion in the rehabilitation plan and in goals set with the patient (Figure 6.3).

- Podiatry referral and footwear reviews need to be considered.

## Mental health issues

- Assessing patients in their own home can be challenging, as establishing a willingness to engage with a physiotherapist may be difficult, due to levels of anxiety or withdrawal.

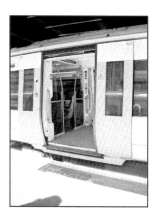

**Figure 6.3** High-level outdoor mobility assessment includes use of public transport.

- If the patient prefers and consents to a familiar person being involved in the assessment process (family, friend, warden, community psychiatric nurse (CPN)) then this may be appropriate.
- Anxiety, depression and dementia all impact on the potential for improvement. The patient may be unable to be proactive in a rehabilitation programme, therefore a more slow-stream approach may need to be offered.
- Patients with chronic cognitive impairment are likely to have limited ability to engage with the rehabilitation programme and medication management; therefore this will need to be taken into account when planning treatment.
- It is essential that there is differentiation of the patient's presentation, for example an acute confusion can be associated with an infection that is treatable (e.g. urinary tract infection).
- Ideally there are effective support networks for patients that can be involved in the implementation of the treatment plan, e.g. community psychiatric nurses, befriending services or clubs (OPG 2005) (Appendix 6.1).

## Reasoning relating to the objective testing for personal and domestic activities of daily living (ADL)

- The functional approach, using the biopsychosocial model is essential when assessing patients in the community.
- Pain, reduced range of movement and/or muscle strength, mobility problems, decreased exercise tolerance due to respiratory and/or cardiac limitations, and mental health issues will become apparent.

### How a patient manages their routine can form part of the baseline assessment

- Examples of how patients organise their routines are:
- Do they use all of their accommodation or do they live in a microenvironment?
- Do they sleep in a bed, a recliner chair or the sofa?
- Are they restricted in moving from lying to sitting to standing?
- Can they access the toilet/commode and manage toileting independently?

- Can they wash and dress themselves?
- Can they prepare hot drinks, light snacks or manage full meal preparation?

- There may already be a package of care in situ to support these tasks, but it is worth considering if improvements can be made.
- Advice/re-education or provision of equipment may be appropriate, if acceptable to the patient. Remember to establish if the person wants to or needs to do the task.
- Patient safety is fundamental and if the patient is not safe with some activities then it is essential that alternatives are found.
- Tele-care systems can reduce risk of problems occurring, with sensors detecting movement from a chair, bed or general activities, such as leaving the bath running or cooker turned on.

## Outcome measures

- All outcome measures need to be carefully documented for consistency.
- Whilst some are validated for use in the community others can and need to be adapted, e.g. the 'Timed up and go' test (TUAG) from the armchair to the front door (Mathias et al 1986).
- Others may be inappropriate due to the limitations in the community setting with space, safety and time, e.g. shuttle walking test (Tobin et al 1999).

## Treatment planning

- Patients are more likely to engage in a treatment programme if there is an obvious benefit to their quality of life, e.g. being able to toilet themselves or make a hot drink.
- In some areas the community occupational therapists offer a 'trusted assessors' course which will provide skills for other professionals to carry out an assessment for basic environmental adaptations, such as simple grab rails, stair rails and chair raises, so that these can be ordered as part of your intervention.
- Environmental changes or adaptations can be offered to improve independence and safety; however, lifestyle choices have to be respected. The patient may wish to live in a cluttered or dirty home. If this has potential to impact on the safety of staff then the physiotherapist has the right to refuse to enter the property. If it is acceptable to the patient, a 'blitz' clean can be offered through the local council, after which health and social care workers may agree to enter the property to carry out the necessary assessments and treatments.
- Documentation of such issues is essential and will ensure that at a later date the initial findings and advice offered can be confirmed (CSP 2000).

## Goal setting and carers

- It is always important to have an indication from the patient of their expectations of treatment.
- This can be achieved through joint goal setting and it is essential that these are negotiated with the patient for realistic treatment plans to be achievable.
- In a community setting this may also involve carers, as the treatment will be carried out within the patient's home environment.

- Consideration needs to be given to:
- The activities are carried out by the carers and why.
- Whether the patient has the ability or desire to take over these tasks.
- Whether the carer/s want this to happen.
- Whether it is appropriate for the carers to be included in the treatment planning.
- Whether the carer/s want this to happen.
- The intensity of the input may affect treatment planning, if the activities need to be supervised to ensure patient safety.
- A domiciliary physiotherapist able to visit once a week will need to plan a different intervention compared to a physiotherapist in an intermediate care team who can arrange for support workers to visit up to three times daily.
- Consideration as to whether the patient needs to be managed in a lesser or greater intensity of service should be part of the assessment process.

## Summary

- This chapter has illustrated how core physiotherapy skills need to be adapted to the community setting.
- The way in which the community physiotherapy service is funded and managed will influence service availability and delivery in different locations.
- However assessment and subsequent treatment should always remain functional, goal-focused and appropriate to the patient and their home environment.

The references for this chapter can be found on www.expertconsult.com.

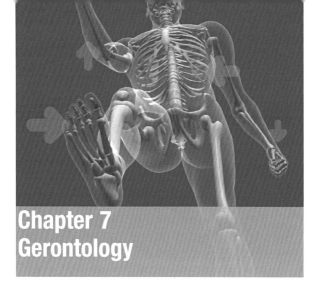

# Chapter 7
# Gerontology

## General principles

- Assessment should be based around the functional ability of the older person and their ability to maintain an independent lifestyle.

- Movement is context-dependent and therefore it is essential to understand the individual's physical and social circumstances and the external environment that indirectly affects the individual.

- Older people are more likely to have a long-term condition, and are also more likely to have impairments resulting from two or more concurrent conditions. The impact of multi-pathology must be taken into account during the assessment process.

- It is important for the physiotherapist to assess whether the presenting problem is due to age-related change, underlying impairments, deconditioning, deskilling or a combination of these. The physiotherapist should also assess the individual's values and beliefs about their health and identify any psychological barriers that may impact on rehabilitation.

- The physiotherapist should include specific assessment of the musculoskeletal, cardiorespiratory and neurological systems depending on the older person's presenting problems. The assessment process may need to accommodate for changes in the older person's ability to participate in a lengthy assessment.

- It may take a number of sessions to complete the assessment.

- Physiotherapy is often part of a multidisciplinary assessment of an older person.

- Teamwork is essential in order to build a comprehensive picture of the older person's abilities and establish an effective treatment plan.

# Knowledge specific to gerontology

## Systemic 'normal' age changes

- The development of age-related changes tends to follow a pattern that is unique to the individual.
- Normal biological ageing progressively lowers the amount of available reserve.
- The rate and extent of decline varies across physiological systems and individuals.
- Physiotherapists should expect greater variability among their older patients.

## Central nervous system: special senses

### Vision

- Visual acuity, accommodation and depth perception decline with age.
- Adaptation to darkness and light occurs more slowly.
- Contrast sensitivity decreases with ageing (Hampton et al 1997).

#### Practical points

- Check that glasses are clean and that the person is wearing the correct pair.
- Ensure that the treatment area is well lit.
- Exercise sheets and information leaflets should be large, bold type.
- Assess the person's ability to distinguish objects in his/her immediate environment.

### Hearing and vestibular system

- Hearing loss especially at higher frequencies is common (Hampton et al 1997).
- The vestibular system shows progressive loss of hair cells, vestibular ganglion cells and nerve fibres which contribute to decline in the ability to detect orientation in space and uncertainty to move around in the dark (Ghosh 1985).

#### Practical points

- Even mild hearing loss makes understanding speech difficult, particularly when there is background noise or more than one person talking.
- Try to reduce background noise as much as possible.
- Face the person to facilitate lip reading.
- Check that hearing aids are switched on.
- If one ear is better, speak on that side.
- Don't shout as this distorts the speech sounds.
- Speak clearly, more slowly and at a slightly lower frequency.
- Sometimes it may be necessary to use written communication (carry some paper with you) or basic sign language.
- Be aware that an older person may come across as confused when in fact they have not heard the question or instruction.

### Skin and somatosensory system

- Older people are less sensitive to:
- Vibration especially in the lower limbs (Kenshalo 1986, Shaffer and Harrison 2007)

- Touch pressure (Wickremaratchi et al 2006)

- Two point discrimination (Shimokata and Kuzuya 1995)

- Cutaneous pain (Lautenbacher et al 2005)

- Smell and taste (Boyce and Shone 2006).

- These changes are due to a reduction in the number and structure of specialised nerve-ending receptors and peripheral nerve degeneration.

- Thinning of the subcutaneous tissue leads to wrinkling of the skin. The skin capillaries bleed more easily.

**Practical points**

- Care should be taken when handling and positioning the older person if they have thin, delicate skin.

- Watch for sensitivity to interventions, e.g. ice, massage.

## Central nervous system: brain and spinal cord

- Ageing is associated with:

- A slow accelerating reduction in brain size with a 10% or greater loss in total brain weight over a normal long life. Both grey and white matter is lost, the former to a greater degree.

- Shrinking of the branches of the dendritic arbour.

- Reductions in the enzymes that help produce neurotransmitters.

- An accumulation of lipofuscin, neurofibrillary tangles and plaques in neurones but not to such a degree as in dementia (Hampton et al 1997).

- A small decline in maximal nerve conduction velocity (Rivner et al 2001).

**Practical points**

- The ability to remember new memories of events or facts, working memory and episodic memory declines in normal ageing (Hedden and Gabrieli, 2004).

- The physiotherapist should supplement instructions with an exercise sheet or visual prompts and instructions.

- The number of exercises may have to be limited and more time given to learn them.

- Changes in nerve conduction velocity do not impact on function.

## Muscles

- Ageing is associated with:

- Loss of muscle mass and a corresponding reduction in maximal muscle strength (Skelton and Beyer 2003, Deschenes 2004).

- Not all muscle groups atrophy at the same rate with weight-bearing muscles showing the most change.

- Loss of motor units and a decreased number of Type II muscle fibres (Proctor et al 1995).

- Slower contraction and more susceptibility to fatigue (Connelly et al 1999).

- Decreased excitability (Porter et al 1994).

- The marked decrease in skeletal muscle strength is due to a combination of biological changes, the accumulation of acute and chronic diseases, reduced physical activity and nutritional deficiencies (Fiatarone and Evans 1993, Doherty 2003).

Practical points

- Performing a task such as rising from a chair may require the frail older person to function near their maximum functional reserve capacity.
- An additional small deficit in muscle function, such as prolonged rest or acute illness, can tip an older person into dependency.
- Appell (1990) found a 3–4% daily reduction in muscle strength during the first week of immobilisation and up to a 40% decrease in isokinetic muscle strength after 3 weeks.
- Muscle atrophy also plays a role in the development of contractures.
- The physiotherapist should encourage the older person to keep as active as possible unless contra-indicated.

## Bones and joints

- Ageing is associated with:
- Universal loss of bone density from about the mid-30s onwards, accelerating after the menopause in women and in the mid-50s in men.
- As we age, the balance between bone formation and re-absorption is upset, leading to a loss over the lifetime (Chan and Duque 2002).
- Excessive cross-linkages makes cartilage less able to handle mechanical stress (Loeser 2004).

Practical points

- Increased stiffness of the connective tissues and degenerative changes in the joints contribute to a decrease in flexibility and range of motion (very small age-related loss) which may affect the ability to execute volitional or compensatory postural responses.

## Gait and posture

- Ageing is associated with:
- Reduced gait speed due to shorter step length and increased time in double stance (Ferrandez et al 1990)
- Reduced hip, knee and ankle movement (Judge et al 1996)
- Increased anterior pelvic tilt (Winter et al 1990)
- Larger degree of out-toeing
- No difference in step width
- No difference in foot clearance
- Increased postural sway (College et al 1994)
- Reduction in height and stooped posture although there are marked variations in older individuals.

Practical points

- The speed an individual chooses for daily ambulation is the most fundamental measure of gait performance.

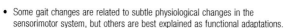

- Some gait changes are related to subtle physiological changes in the sensorimotor system, but others are best explained as functional adaptations.
- Older people may unconsciously choose to walk in a manner that increases the proportion of time spent in stance and double support to increase stability.

## Respiratory system

- Age-related changes begin slowly after the third decade but progress more rapidly after the sixth decade. Changes over time are a combination of biological factors (age-related), environmental factors (pollution) and personal/social factors (smoking).
- Ageing is associated with:
- Increased stiffness of the chest wall
- Decreased strength of intercostals and accessory muscles of respiration
- Enlarged alveolar ducts/alveoli
- Decreased elasticity and increased cross-linked collagen
- Increased functional reserve and closing capacity
- Decreased local pulmonary vascular regulation
- Reduced chemoreceptor and muscle response
- Reduced effectiveness of cilia (Hampton et al 1997).

**Practical points**

- Despite these changes, the respiratory system is capable of maintaining adequate oxygenation and ventilation during the entire lifespan.
- However, the respiratory system reserve reduces with age, and diminished ventilatory response to hypoxia and hypercapnia makes older people more vulnerable to respiratory failure during high demand states, e.g. heart failure, pneumonia.

## Cardiovascular system

- Ageing is associated with:
- An increase in heart weight
- Thickening of the endocardium and the semilunar and atrioventricular valves
- Stiffening of the artery walls
- Increased peripheral vascular resistance
- A decrease in cardiac output
- A decrease in heart rate and maximal heart rate (Hampton et al 1997).

**Practical points**

- The ageing heart can significantly increase its maximum output and allows older people to perform vigorous exercise, although not up to the same intensity as a younger individual.

## Autonomic nervous system

- Ageing is associated with:
- Abnormal central and peripheral thermoregulatory responses leading to reduced ability to regulate body temperature (Kenney and Munce 2003).

GERONTOLOGY

7

**Practical points**

- Extra precautions should be taken during strenuous exercise and hot conditions.

## Genitourinary system

- Ageing is associated with:
- A decrease in weight and volume of the kidney (20–30% by age 90)
- Reduction in glomeruli by up to 50% over the lifespan
- A decrease in proximal tubule volume and length
- Reduction in bladder capacity
- Loss of muscle tone resulting in difficulty in emptying the bladder or in some cases involuntary loss of urine (Hampton et al 1997)
- The ageing kidney has a lowered reserve. Kidney disease or acute illness can have serious effects on renal function.

## Gastrointestinal system

- Ageing is associated with:
- Reduction in the intestinal mucosa blood flow
- Atrophy of the musculature of the intestinal wall
- Reduction in vitamin and iron absorption (Hampton et al 1997)
- The gastrointestinal system functions well in healthy older people
- However dietary neglect, disease and medication may lead to an altered nutritional status.

## Recognising delirium

- Delirium (acute confusional state) is a common condition in older people affecting up to 30% of medical (Siddiqi et al 2006) and up to 50% post fractured neck of femur patients (Marcantonio 2000).
- Delirium is characterised by an acute (hours to days), fluctuating change in mental status with inattention and altered levels of consciousness.
- There are two main types:
- Hyperactive delirium: agitation and visual hallucinations
- Hypoactive delirium: lethargy and withdrawal.
- There are many precipitating factors including immobility, malnutrition, intercurrent illness, dehydration and stress of admission to hospital or other unfamiliar settings (Elie et al 1998).
- It is important that the physiotherapist is able to recognise the signs of delirium and feedback to the MDT.
- Symptoms generally resolve when the underlying cause is treated.

## Adapting assessment of older people with cognitive impairment

- Poor memory means that history taking is often difficult and to obtain a clear idea of the presenting problem may take time.
- Older people with cognitive impairment may not be able to recall how long they have had a physical problem or pain.

- The physiotherapist needs to recognise confabulation – filling in gaps in their memory with false memories.
- Information may have to be supplemented by a family member or a person that knows them well.
- Initial approach:
- Approach the person slowly from the front
- Respect personal space
- Address the person by name and make eye contact
- Keep hand and body movement smooth and unhurried
- Speak clearly, in a manner acceptable to an adult
- Make use of facial expression
- Be courteous.
- Verbal strategies:
- Give the person plenty of time
- Use short sentences
- Limit requests to one at a time
- Use repetition, and change wording if necessary
- Experiment with words and expressions
- Avoid inviting a refusal
- Use word requests in a positive way
- Give step-by-step instructions
- Use word requests for an automatic response
- Use tone of voice to suggest the ease of the task
- Watch the person's reactions to requests.
- When there are two therapists attending the person, only one should speak (Oddy 2003).
- The timing of the assessment can affect the outcome.
- Greater accuracy is likely if the activity is carried out at the appropriate time of the day, e.g. bed transfers assessed in the morning rather than the afternoon.
- Remember to gain insight into night time by asking carers and/or nursing staff.
- The assessment of activities such as walking also needs special consideration since the level of performance may be variable through the day.
- The physiotherapist should assess the older person at different times in order to measure the extent of these variations.

## Subjective assessment: where information may be found and the level of detail required

- Information sources: patient, next of kin, carers, medical records, 'passports': e.g. learning difficulties, dementia, health and social care records (IT systems), other health care professionals involved in the care of the older person, such as district nurse, community matron, community psychiatric nurse (CPN).

- An older person may report abuse. Reassure the person and ensure that you are aware of the safeguarding of older adults policy, so you know what procedures you should follow.
- Cognition: be aware of the person's orientation to place, person and time. In the acute hospital environment, the doctors and/or occupational therapists may perform cognitive screening tests, e.g. Abbreviated Mental Test Score (AMTS) or Mini Mental State Examination (MMSE)
- AMTS: scored out of 10. A score of less than 7 indicates some cognitive impairment
- MMSE/Folstein: scored out of 30. A score ≥25 points is effectively normal (intact). Below this, scores can indicate severe (≤9 points), moderate (10–20 points) or mild (21–24 points) cognitive impairment.
- Mood: be aware of the person's level of engagement during the subjective assessment.
- Red flags include:
- Sadness
- Fatigue
- Abandoning or losing interest in hobbies or other pleasurable pastimes
- Social withdrawal and isolation
- Weight loss and/or loss of appetite
- Sleep disturbances
- Loss of self-worth
- Increased use of alcohol or other drugs
- Fixation on death; suicidal thoughts or attempts
- Unexplained or aggravated aches and pains
- Lack of interest in personal care (missing meals, neglecting personal hygiene, forgetting medications)
- Memory problems.

## History of the present condition

- What movement difficulties are they experiencing, how long ago was it that they were able to do the particular activity (days, weeks, months) and what do they think is stopping them?
- If the person finds it difficult to remember what activities are difficult, asking about their normal daily routine may be helpful.
- What does the person understand by their condition?

## Pain

- Ask the older person if they have any pain at rest or on movement.
- Use a range of alternative words to describe pain, e.g. sore, aching
- Ask about the nature, location and intensity of pain
- Ask about impact on functional abilities and participation
- Ask the person to locate the pain either by asking them to point to the area on themselves or use a pain map/body chart
- Use standardised scales in a format that is accessible to the individual.

- Self-report assessment scales such as the Numerical Rating Scale (NRS) and the Verbal Rating Scale (VRS) are recommended (Concise Guidance to Good Practice Number 8: The assessment of pain in older people (RCP 2007)).

## Specific questions on falls history

- How many slips, trips or falls in the last 12 months?
- Include the descriptors of slips and trips as some older people may consider a trip as insignificant. If it was a slip or trip, clarify what exactly caused it?
- What was the individual doing at the time of the fall? A detailed history is essential, including location of the fall.
- Did anyone witness the fall?
- What injuries were sustained as a result of the fall? Does the pattern of injury described and/or seen fit with the details of the fall?
- Watch for those who have sustained black eyes or facial bruising/fractures. Facial injuries may result from falls due to syncope (Wade et al 2004).
- Was the individual able to get up from the floor? How did they summon help? Many older people do not injure themselves in a fall, but are unable to get up from the floor and may stay on the floor for some time (Wild et al 1981, Vellas et al 1987, Tinetti et al 1993).
- Any loss of consciousness? Again this suggests a medical reason for falling.
- Any signs/symptoms before the fall? Ask the person to describe the symptoms.
- Dizziness is a common symptom.
- Many different feelings can be described as dizziness.
- Vertigo is often described as a spinning sensation. The person may feel that they are moving or that the surroundings are moving while they remain still. Vertigo usually occurs when a person is standing but can occur while sitting, lying down, or changing position. People with vertigo may also have nausea, sometimes with vomiting, and nystagmus. Benign paroxysmal positional vertigo (BPPV) is a common cause of dizziness in older people. Symptoms are almost always precipitated by a change in head position, e.g. getting out of bed or rolling over in bed.
- Presyncope is often described as a feeling of light-headedness, generalised weakness and a sense of 'going down'. It can be cardiogenic, e.g. arrhythmia or situational. Older people may report light-headedness or faintness after moving from supine to standing or sitting to standing that can occur up to 5 minutes after the change in position (Craig 1994). Numerous diseases have been found to be associated, including heart failure, Type 1 diabetes, Parkinson's disease, stroke, dementia and depression (Mathias 1995, Tivlis et al 1996). The physiotherapist needs to be alert to small clues, e.g.: reluctance to walk or participate in any activity that requires an upright posture, sitting down hurriedly or becoming pale on standing.
- Dysequilibrium is a sense of unsteadiness or loss of balance. The person may feel that they need to hold onto something to maintain their balance.
- Fear of falling: are there any activities that they avoid or are concerned about performing? Fear of falling is prevalent among community-dwelling older people and may be independent of fall injuries or previous falls (Howland et al 1998, Bruce et al 2002). Prospective studies have shown that fear of falling predicts deterioration in physical function, decreased activity and admission into care homes (Cummings et al 2000, Vellas et al 1996).

- Fear of falling is a predictor of falls (Mendes de Leon et al 1996, Delbaere et al 2010). Fear of falling may impact on the older person's participation in physiotherapy assessment and intervention.

## Past medical history

- Identifying pre-existing disease that may be contributing to risk of falling and/or functional problems is an important component in physiotherapy assessment.

- Lower limb problems, e.g. osteoarthritis of the hip or knee with muscle wasting of associated muscle groups, reduced range of movement and pain has a detrimental effect on postural stability and has been shown to increase risk of falls (Sturnieks et al 2004, Arden et al 2006).

- Neurological disease that affects muscle power, balance, gait, sensation or ability to plan and execute locomotor activities will impact both on functional performance and falls risk.

- CVA, Parkinson's disease and peripheral neuropathy have been associated with an increased risk of falls (Burns 1994, Richardson and Hurvitz 1995, Herndon et al 1997, Jorgensen et al 2002, Allcock et al 2009).

- Urinary incontinence, frequency, nocturia and rushing to the toilet to avoid incontinence are associated with increased risk of falls and fractures (Brown et al 2000, Chiarelli et al 2009).

- Cognitive impairment and dementia increase the risk of falls and fractures (Kallin et al 2005).

- The most common types of dementia are:

- Alzheimer's disease: gradual onset of memory impairment including disorientation to time and place, difficulty with abstract thinking and familiar tasks, poor or decreased judgement. Gait and balance impairment occur in the later stages of disease.

- Multi-infarct dementia: stepwise progression with focal neurological signs and symptoms and memory impairment.

- Lewy body dementia: progressive memory impairment, visual hallucinations, fluctuations in autonomic processes, signs of parkinsonism (tremor, rigidity, festinating gait), recurrent falls.

- Visual impairment such as cataracts, macular degeneration and glaucoma exacerbate age-related visual loss and thereby decrease postural stability and increase falls risk (Ivers et al 1998, Wood et al 2009). Use of multifocals has been reported to increase falls risk as the near-vision lenses impair distance contrast sensitivity and depth perception in the lower visual field (Lord et al 2002).

- Any previous fragility and fractures?

## Drug history

- Note medication prescribed.
- How does the older person manage their medications?
- Research shows that the greater the number of medications (four or more) taken the greater the risk of falls (Lipsitz et al 1991, Leipzig et al 1999a, 1999b).

- Polypharmacy increases the risk of drug interactions as well as adverse reactions which include confusion, fatigue, urinary incontinence, constipation and orthostatic hypotension (Monane and Avorn 1996).

- Some medications have been associated with increased risk of falls. These include antidepressants, antipsychotics, anticonvulsants and benzodiazepines (Ensrud et al 2003).

- Some medications can impair mobility, e.g. antipsychotics, benzodiazepines, anticonvulsants (Robin et al 1996). The physiotherapist might be the first person to link impaired gait with the older person's medications.

- An individual might not report or recall all of their medical conditions. Knowledge of medications will give you important information about a person's medical history.

- If you are working in a hospital, each ward will have a British National Formulary (BNF) which provides practical information on medications.

## Social history

- Accommodation:
- Lives alone?
- Detail of access into and within the property
- Stairs/steps and position of rails
- Equipment already in situ, e.g. bed lever, riser recliner chair, raised toilet seat
- Location of rooms.
- Formal and informal networks plus frequency/adequacy of support/ sustainability:
- Always consider the health of an informal carer, their lifestyle and other responsibilities.
- An older person may be admitted to hospital not because of deterioration in their own condition, but because of a change in the health or circumstances of their carer.
- Exercise tolerance:
- Distances walked and level of assistance required, outdoor mobility
- Use of walking aids, what, why and for how long?
- Ability to climb stairs
- Ability to use public transport.
- Care home resident:
- Care homes may send a transfer summary or a 'passport' with the older person if they come to hospital which can provide a useful insight to function.
- Make contact with the care home and confirm normal level of function with a named staff member.
- Confirm whether the care home is residential or nursing.
- Clarify whether there has been a change in function and the time frame of change.
- The staff member may report specific functional difficulties which can help you focus your assessment.

- Use of alcohol:
- Be aware that some older people may have been dependent upon alcohol during their life; also a group of older people who begin to drink excessively for the first time in old age (O'Connell et al 2003).
- Patients frequently do not volunteer this information or may deny it if questioned directly.
- Any previous physiotherapy intervention and outcome?

## Reasoning behind the choice of objective testing or measurements to be carried out and tips on how best to apply these

- Tests of everyday functional ability should be appropriate to the older person's ability level and needs which have been established by subjective history taking.
- In practice, older people will need to attempt many of the same daily activities such as getting out of bed, rising from a chair, standing and walking including walking outside or across a road.
- The tests should be started at a level which allows achievement of the test.
- The sequence should be halted before failure seems certain.
- If success is in doubt, help should be provided and sufficient time to give the person opportunity to succeed.
- If the person varies in performance from day to day, or morning from evening, tests should be repeated on several occasions to get a fuller picture.
- For a frail person, the tests may need to be conducted over several sessions.
- Choose procedures that capture the most information with the least number of activities.
- Muscle weakness correlates with several measures of functional status (Skelton et al 1994). Assessment of sit to stand will provide important information on functional ROM, muscle strength, exercise tolerance and balance that may be more relevant to identifying functional problems than traditional ROM and muscle strength assessment.

## Objective assessment: tools or techniques specific to older people

- Observation:
- Level of alertness and posture
- Muscle bulk, skin condition, condition of hands, nails, teeth and clothing
- Older people with very severe cognitive/communication impairment may not be able to self-report pain. Look for behavioural responses such as facial expression, change in body movements and activity patterns, change in mental status, e.g. confusion, aggression, or autonomic changes such as pallor or tachycardia. Assessment should include insight from carers and/or family members to interpret the meanings of their behaviours.

- Upper limbs:
- ROM similar to that of young people. Minor degrees of limitation may not affect function.
- Screen ROM by asking the older person to raise their hands over their head and behind their back. Further MSK assessment may be indicated.
- Feel muscle tone.
- Rigidity may be most easily detected at the elbow and wrist.
- Outstretched hands: assess for tremor and drift of the limb.
- Lower limbs:
- ROM similar to that of younger people. Further MSK assessment may be indicated.
- Feel muscle tone.
- Contractures develop quickly if immobile for a short period or the older person spends the greater part of the day in a chair.
- Muscle strength: in sitting
- Test hip flexors/abductors, quadriceps, ankle muscles.
- In large prospective studies, reduced quadriceps strength has been found to increase the risk of falls and fractures (Campbell et al 1989, Nguyen et al 1993, Lord et al 1994).
- Lower limb strength muscle weakness has also been found to be associated with falls, particularly the knee and ankle muscles (Tinetti et al 1993, Whipple et al 1987, Nevitt et al 1989, Studenski et al 1991, Wolfson et al 1995).
- Feet and footwear: Ask the older person to remove their socks
- This will give you information about flexibility and dexterity as well as observing condition of skin, nails, callous formation and deformities.
- Foot problems are a contributing factor to mobility impairment in older people. Older people with painful feet walk more slowly (Guralnik et al 1994) and have more difficulty performing ADLs (Benvenutti et al 1995). An Australian cross-sectional study found that foot problems were associated with impaired balance and function as well as history of multiple falls (Menz and Lord 2001).
- Examine footwear for signs of wear.
- Balance: what activities does the older person need to do?
- Sitting: what support is required to maintain balance?
- Can the patient sit unsupported with both feet on the floor?
- How long can they maintain this position?
- What degree of independent activity can be carried out?
- Standing: what support is required to maintain balance?
- Can the patient stand unsupported?
- How long can they maintain standing?
- What degree of independent activity can be carried out?
- Do they widen or change the base of support?
- Do they use their hands for support?

- Transfers: observe the pattern of movement, speed, quality and safety plus ease of the task.
- Do they weight bear more on one leg?
- Do they position one leg behind the other?
- Do they use their hands?
- Do they widen or change the base of support?
- Document the height of the chair and bed that you are assessing from. Is this similar to the home environment?
- Gait: If possible, analyse gait as the patient walks into the treatment room, within their property or around the bedside.
- Consider the environment especially in the acute setting (the familiarity of home, use of furniture, different floor coverings). Initiation of walking, presence of freezing, ability to start and stop (any hesitation).
- Locomotion: width of base, foot clearance, arm swing, step length, step timing, variability of stepping, weight transfer, heel strike, head position, general posture
- Quality and safety of turning
- Reactions if imbalance occurs
- Use of walking aid and appropriateness
- Exercise tolerance
- Ability to walk outdoors including kerbs, slopes, uneven ground, use of public transport, getting in and out of a car
- Steps and stairs. An older person may need to be able to negotiate steps/stairs in other properties rather than their own
- Obstacles.
- Dual tasking: is the older person able to walk and talk? There is growing evidence that gait changes in dual task conditions are associated with an increased risk of falls (Beauchet et al 2008).
- Frail older people have been shown to stop walking when they start a conversation with a walking companion (Lundin-Olsson et al 1997).

## Treatment planning: based on subjective and objective assessment findings

- Identify the physical and any psychological impairments contributing to the functional problem.
- Consider the extent to which each factor is limiting the older person's ability to function and the degree to which physiotherapy can modify each factor.
- Rank the problems in order of priority.
- Ask the older person:
- 'What are the most important tasks that you will need to do to look after yourself (by yourself/help from carer)?'
- 'Right now, which of these tasks are you NOT confident that you will be able to do?'
- Focus on a small number of problems.
- Empower the older person to set their own goals.
- Make sure that you discuss their potential for improvement.

- Sometimes the physiotherapist may need to consider the goals of the family/caregiver.
- Be aware that the older person's goals and the caregiver's and/or physiotherapist's idea of what is safe to achieve may be different.
- In these cases, consider the individual's rights and their capacity to take risks.
- The physiotherapist's role is to highlight the risks and try to minimise them as much as possible.

The references for this chapter can be found on www.expertconsult.com.

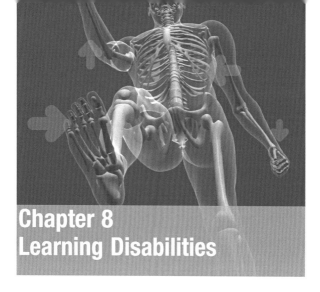

# Chapter 8
# Learning Disabilities

## Introduction

- People with learning disabilities (LD) will meet with all sorts of health professionals in all types of settings, from GP practices, outpatient clinics, general hospital inpatient wards and specialist clinics.

- This volume will address some of the difficulties, and issues faced by physiotherapists when assessing people with LD, whether in the generic or specialist services.

- Reference will be made to the legislation in the United Kingdom, e.g. 'Valuing people (DOH, 2001) and 'The same as you' (Scottish Executive 2000).

- The 'Death by indifference' report by Mencap (2007) highlighted six case studies where the National Health Service (NHS) failed to meet the needs of people with LD in general hospital settings, with the neglect resulting in unnecessary suffering and premature death.

- Three of the patients included in the case studies had chest complications, which were inadequately treated by physiotherapy.

- The report emphasised that the following health inequalities were experienced by people with LD and which need to be addressed:

- People with LD were not a priority for the NHS

- Many health care professionals do not understand how to work with LD

- Health care professionals did not listen to family and carers

- Health care professionals did not understand the law around capacity and consent

- Health care professionals rely inappropriately on their own estimates of a person with LD.

# What is a learning disability (LD)?

- LD is not a disease and is not an illness and will be evident from childhood, and In many cases without a clear cause.
- There are often links with pre- or postnatal injury or disease.
- There may also be links with genetics, chromosomal abnormalities or environmental factors.
- There is a historical perspective to LD which has resulted in people being excluded, institutionalised, labelled and deprived of their rights (Barrell 2007).
- The World Health Organization (1992) has defined learning disabilities as, 'a state of arrested or incomplete development of mind'.
- LD is generally understood to be a combination of the following:
- An intellectual impairment
- Impaired social functioning
- Identified early onset with an impact on development.
- LD can be divided into four very basic groups based on IQ scores:
- Mild       IQ score of 50 to 70
- Moderate   IQ score of 35 to 50
- Severe     IQ score of 20 to 30
- Profound   IQ score of less than 20.
- Those people with moderate or severe LD may also display other associated physical and mental health problems.

## Prevalence of LD and profound and multiple learning disability (PMLD)

- The British Institute of Learning Disabilities (www.bild.org.uk), estimates that there are 1.2 million people with LD in the UK.
- According to research completed at Lancaster University (Emerson and Hatton 2005), approximately 985 000 people in England had a LD, around about 2% of the general population.
- Approximately 796 000 of these are over the age of 20. It was estimated that there were 21 000 people with PMLD.
- From Scottish statistics there is an indication that about 2–4% of the population have LD.
- The number of adults with LD is predicted to increase by 11% between the years 2001 to 2021 (Emerson and Hatton 2005).
- The prevalence of LD in the population over the age of 60 is predicted to increase by 36% from 2001 to 2021.

## Profound and multiple learning disability

- The term PMLD is used to identify people with LD and additional disabilities.
- People with PMLD form a small, but significant section of the wider population of people with LD.
- Carnaby (2004) highlighted a difference of opinion relating to terminology.

- The definitions of profound intellectual disability most often cited include having an IQ of below 20 and describing individuals as those who are severely limited in their ability to understand or comply with requests or instructions. Most such individuals are immobile or severely restricted in mobility, incontinent, and capable at most of only the rudimentary forms of non-verbal communication (WHO 1992).

- People with PMLD are likely to be more vulnerable and require additional support with healthcare management, mobility and continence and the consequential outcomes.

- In practice, people with PMLD may learn to function within their environment using a variety of communication strategies.

## Challenging behaviour

- There are specific conditions that can predispose an individual to display challenging behaviour.

- Emerson (1995) defined challenging behaviours as being 'culturally abnormal behaviours(s) of such intensity, frequency or duration that the physical safety of the person or others is likely to be placed in serious jeopardy'.

- A further definition states: 'behaviour which is likely to seriously limit use of or result in the person being denied access to, ordinary community facilities.'

- Types of challenging behaviour can be described as: aggression, self-injury, destructiveness, over activity, inappropriate social or sexual conduct, bizarre mannerisms or eating inappropriate objects.

## Autism

- The concept of autism is broad, with it being described as a spectrum disorder.

- It can present as a subtle problem of social understanding and functioning or as profoundly severe disabilities.

- People on the spectrum are referred to as having autistic spectrum disorder (ASD) or in the absence of LD and in the upper regions of the intellectual quotient of the spectrum (IQ > 70) are defined as having Asperger's syndrome.

- People with LD may therefore exhibit autistic tendencies.

- Wing and Gould (1979) proposed that all people on the autism spectrum, irrespective of their cognition, have a triad of key impairments, which are:

- Communication – including language impairment across all modes of communication from speech, intonation, gesture, facial expression and other body language.

- Imagination involving rigidity and inflexibility of thought process, resistance to change, obsessional and ritualistic behaviour.

- Socialisation – such as difficulties with social relationships, poor social timing, lack of social empathy, rejection of normal body contact, inappropriate eye contact.

- It is important for a physiotherapist to have an awareness of the effects of autism if linked to a person with LD, so that an approach can be appropriately adapted and an intervention designed to meet their individual needs.

## Legislation

### Mental Capacity Act (2005)

- The mental capacity act is relevant to physiotherapy as it covers the issues of consent and capacity.
- This is particularly pertinent for people with LD and the treatment they receive.
- It is a fundamental principle that people have the right to determine what happens to their body.
- This right is reflected in the rules of professional conduct and standards of physiotherapy practice (CSP 2005a).
- People with LD in the past have not necessarily been involved in decision-making and often professionals and carers may not have considered whether they have the capacity to make decisions.
- As physiotherapists, it is important to remember that touching a patient prior to obtaining valid consent may constitute battery under civil or criminal law.
- Gaining an individual's consent to assessment and treatment is more than a legal requirement; it is a matter of common courtesy and helps to establish a relationship of trust and confidence (CSP 2005b).
- Capacity must be assessed for each individual task, e.g. someone may be able to consent to aquatic physiotherapy by being at and seeing the pool and they consent by changing and coming to the pool area. However they may lack capacity to consent to a smear test or understand the consequences of not undertaking the test.
- Each situation has to be assessed individually and it cannot be assumed someone 'has capacity or not' as it depends on the nature of the task or demand.

### Mental Health Act (2005)

- The Mental Health Act has provided a legal framework to protect vulnerable people.
- The act is underpinned by five key principles:
- A presumption of capacity – every adult has the right to make his or her own decisions and must be assumed to have capacity unless it is proved otherwise
- The right for individuals to be supported to make their own decisions
- That individuals must retain the right to make what might seem as eccentric or unwise decisions
- Best interest
- Least restrictive intervention.

## Knowledge specific to learning disability

### Multi-disciplinary team (MDT)/multiagency working

- Physiotherapists working in the field of LD rarely work in isolation.
- They are generally based in a MDT made up of a variety of health care professionals; including specialist LD nurses, occupational therapists, speech and language therapists, psychologists and psychiatrists.

- Joint working is carried out with a number of professionals depending on the needs of the client.
- Close work also takes place with the care management team who are either social workers or occasionally LD nurses.
- Although some individuals live at home with family providing the main care, many individuals live in supported accommodation and therefore close working is essential with the care providers and local authority day services.
- Carers have either very limited medical knowledge or none at all.
- This is something that all physiotherapists should bear in mind when giving advice or training these staff.

## Communication

- Many physiotherapists consider themselves to have excellent communication skills, but the usual verbal or written skills may be of limited use with someone who has LD.
- Working with this client group requires skills in both the delivery of information and comprehension of verbal and non-verbal messages.
- Speech and language therapists (SALT) can be a valuable source of information and there are courses available to gain a grounding in augmentative communication skills.
- However, courses are not always immediately accessible and therefore the skills need to be developed in light of increased awareness over time.
- It is often easy to make assumptions about someone's level of comprehension as many individuals develop ways of interpreting their environment, such as situational cues, where routine may play a part in understanding a message, e.g. asking someone if they want a drink, when you are holding a cup of tea, or asking someone if they want to go out, when you have their coat in your hand.
- The question itself may not be understood, but by holding a cup or coat the message is reinforced.
- Many clients use such 'objects of reference' to communicate or use simple signing.
- As individuals with LD may have no verbal communication, it is necessary to develop skills in other forms of communication and these are many and diverse.
- Individuals may express pain and discomfort in a variety of ways and skills in reading body language and facial expression need to be developed.
- Alternatively increased symptoms may be expressed through an increase in what may appear to be 'challenging behaviours'.
- Physiotherapists are often dependent on carers in these situations to describe changes in someone's behaviour and from there a clear picture may emerge as to what is affecting the individual.
- For example; if an individual is uncomfortable in their seating, this may be expressed by self-injurious behaviour, as they may not be able to change their position to relieve pressure.
- They are reliant on others to interpret their need.
- When working with a diverse range of professionals and unqualified carers both written and verbal skills are essential and the ability to translate 'jargon'

into easily understood language is necessary as carers assist with assessments and/or implementation of physiotherapy programmes.

- It is essential to ensure that carers are able to understand what is being said and what is required in order for the individual to receive the best management for their problems.

## Conditions and diagnoses

- With advances in medicine generally, there are a number of specific conditions where in the past individuals rarely lived beyond childhood and therefore as they become adults, knowledge of how the condition presents is unknown. As a result physiotherapy management is difficult to predict requiring skills in treating the presenting symptom/s.

- Physiotherapists tend to work holistically with LD clients, which means they rarely treat a specific ailment or injury in isolation.

- People with LD may of course sustain injuries or experience conditions similar to the general population, therefore a knowledge of working with fractures, low back pain, arthritis, respiratory conditions and any clinical area in which physiotherapists work is necessary.

- Conditions need to be assessed and treated in relation to the individual's LD, primary diagnosis if they have one and any challenging behaviour present, e.g.:

- Clients with Down's syndrome presenting with early-onset dementia, their general lax ligaments will have an effect on safe handling as they require increased physical assistance.

- Individuals with cerebral palsy as they reach the fourth or fifth decade of life present with similar physical deterioration as post-poliomyelitis. This needs to be taken into account when planning for future accommodation needs.

- Wheelchair-dependent clients may develop osteoporosis through lack of weight bearing and many other individuals may develop osteoporosis as a side effect of various medications.

- Side effects of medications may lead to development of Parkinson-type symptoms.

- Eating and drinking difficulties and dysphagia may develop in relation to the ageing process of cerebral palsy or dementia, where joint working with the speech and language therapist around appropriate posture and positioning takes place.

- Altered 'body shape' (e.g. scoliosis) resulting in poor respiratory function, pain and discomfort and decreased mobility.

## Epilepsy

- 21% of people with a learning disability experience epilepsy, which increases to 50% with a diagnosis of cerebral palsy (Rennie 2007).

- Epilepsy has a profound effect on an individual's emotional, social and physical wellbeing, with seizures types varying from absences, myoclonic jerks, tonic–clonic and atonic, to more complex types.

- All of these can impact on a physiotherapy assessment and treatment programme, however, epilepsy should not be seen as a reason to avoid treatments such as aquatic or rebound therapy.

## Transition

- Clients are usually accepted onto a caseload when in transition from the paediatric service and will remain within the adult LD team until the end of their life.

- In a special school, physiotherapy provision tends to be routine and therefore children are seen regularly.

- Many children with disabilities tend to access mainstream schools today, where they may only see a physiotherapist once a term or even annually at a medical review and therefore their physical presentation when they leave school and enter adult services may not be the optimum.

- Older children in the latter years of schooling may not consider physiotherapy a priority in their lives. The result can be that an individual's physiotherapy needs are greater in the initial transition phase.

- Good communication skills may be required to explain the nature of an individual's likely deterioration in skills and function and therefore the need for intervention. This explanation is often required not only to the individual themselves, but to family members and carers.

- Part of the role of the physiotherapist working with LD may be to facilitate services from primary care.

- Physiotherapists working in the acute sector may often feel unable to treat people with LD in a hospital situation, perhaps due to an inability to communicate effectively or a lack of knowledge and experience of working with individuals with a LD or challenging behaviour.

- If an individual is admitted to hospital following a CVA or a fracture for example, treatment and mobilisation to ensure a safe discharge may result in reduced levels of mobility and function which will need to be regained once the individual has been discharged home.

## Approach to assessment

- Physiotherapists are trained to assess patients using specific assessment tools that tend to follow a set process, with each component of the assessment being carried out in a specific order.

- In non-LD practice a diagnosis is usually available prior to any assessment, therefore clinical reasoning can start before the individual is seen and treatment options considered in advance.

- With LD there is often no clear clinical diagnosis and therefore the physiotherapist may have no idea in advance of how the individual may present and therefore no opportunity to prepare specific assessment tools or interventions.

- The physiotherapists will need to be open-minded and flexible in order to effectively assess and treat someone with LD.

- A diagnosis of cerebral palsy does not indicate whether an individual is mobile with a mild hemiplegia, diplegic using a walking aid, independently mobile using a wheelchair or presenting with a profound and multiple disability.

- Similarly, a diagnosis of mild, moderate or severe LD gives no indication of an individual's level of communication or physical ability.

- It is essential that additional information is obtained from the referrer about an individual's general presentation before an assessment is considered.

127

## History

- Due to potential communication difficulties it is often not possible to gain a history directly from the individual themselves.
- Therefore this information should be gained in advance (where possible) from family members, carers, case/care manager and other appropriate professionals.
- However, it should be borne in mind that different carers might have different perceptions about an individual's past history or history of the presenting condition.

## Assessment

- Due to a potentially limited attention span or behavioural difficulties, the time available for the assessment may be shorter than necessary and it may not be possible to complete the assessment in one go.
- The assessment may need to be carried out over two or more sessions. Therefore, it may be necessary to carry out the assessment on more than one visit and this may happen as a result of seeing the individual in unfamiliar surroundings or with different carers or for no obvious reason.
- Previous discussion with the referrer and/or carers, can help the physiotherapist to know what structure will be required and what assessment tools may be useful.
- As much of the assessment as possible should be carried out through observation and it is necessary to retain information or be able to write brief notes, as it is not always possible to write things down at the time.
- At least one further visit is often required to fill in any blanks that may have been missed out on previous visits.

### Examples of different approaches to assessment

- Knowledge about a mobile client can be gained about their gait pattern, weight-bearing and muscle power, as they walk into the assessment area.
- It should not be necessary to ask the individual to specifically perform these tasks and indeed they may not understand why this would be required.
- Discreet observation can be carried out as a client mobilises around a familiar environment, without them being aware that they are being formally assessed.
- This alternative gathering of information can help to provide an insight into someone's mobility levels and possible influences of pain.
- If a client is wheelchair-dependent, information about their sitting balance and seated posture can be gained straight away through observation alone.
- That an individual is assisted to transfer using a hoist will in itself give information about their ability to weight bear or transfer. The type of hoist or sling used can provide further insight, e.g. if an individual is transferred with a full sling, this indicates increased dependence and possible poor trunk control, whereas to use a 'dress' sling (occasionally described as a toileting sling), an individual must have a degree of trunk and upper limb control.
- The type of sling can also give information about an individual's continence as it requires more than one transfer to access a toilet if a full sling is used for transfers.

- If specific measurements of joint range are required, it may be necessary to enlist the support of a carer. This could be due to potential behavioural issues and/or the positive way a client relates to a particular carer.

- Discussing the assistance someone requires for personal care or how easy or difficult it is to assist someone to wash or dress can indicate any limitation in their hip or shoulder movements.

- The exact number of degrees of movement is rarely necessary as a general range for functional purposes is more often what is required.

- It is also important to consider who the assessment is for and why? Working as part of the MDT and also as part of an integrated team, which may include care managers, may lead to a number of requests for assessments for different reasons.

- Initial assessments may entail the physiotherapist carrying out an assessment identifying the appropriateness of the team referral and identification of specific assessment needs.

- Commissioners are involving physiotherapists and other members of the MDT in assessments for continuing care, with this process often being a joint procedure.

- Care managers may request assessments to establish levels of mobility and this can help formulate appropriate plans in respect of the person's housing needs, day service needs and/or residential placement.

- Moving and handling assessments will be required to reduce risk of injury to carers and clients.

## Subjective information

- The physiotherapist has access to a 'toolbox' of assessments that can be adapted for use in LD.

- Barrell (2007) suggested that LD physiotherapists do not use a uniform assessment process because there is no single tool that would meet the needs of the individual.

- Barrell further suggests this is because LD is 'not a single medical condition with identifiable boundaries'.

- No two individuals with LD will have the same presenting features and problems.

- Even with known genetic conditions the variability within a group can be quite extensive.

- The range of abilities, disabilities and cognitive impairment can be vast, therefore any objective measurement has to be sensitive enough to be able to pick up on this variation.

- The student or junior physiotherapist coming into LD must therefore have a good basic knowledge of the more common genetic conditions and some of the likely problems that individuals may face and are referred to physiotherapy for; for example conditions with low muscle tone or lax ligaments such as Prader–Willi and Down's syndromes.

- The problems associated with the condition can be further compounded by weight problems.

- It is important not to get bogged down in the specific diagnosis and common presenting factors of known genetic conditions, believing it is important to know them all. It is more helpful to have access to good reference texts on genetic conditions and refer to them as necessary.

- It is more important to be able to recognise what the problem is and be able to assess and treat it.
- It is important that everyone recognises that individuals with LD are at the same risk of any of the secondary conditions and problems as faced by the general population.
- Barrell (2007) describes some of the assessment tools that can be used with LD, with many of these being geared towards measuring someone's abilities and function.
- They can be quite subjective, e.g. goal attainment scoring, where the physiotherapist who is familiar with the individual sets the goals for that person and then these are reassessed. The goals are therefore very client-specific and the time scales can be chosen by the client/carer and physiotherapist.
- As with most assessments of individuals with LD these formats rely on the physiotherapist having an in-depth knowledge of the client.
- History taking may not involve the client directly, with information being provided by families, carers and other agencies.
- Some clients have large files going back to the days of long-stay hospitals and there is a danger that the history passed down may be based on hearsay and preconceived ideas.

## Objective testing

- Some valid reliable objective measurement tools can be applied to LD, e.g. the modified Ashworth Scale for assessing tone (Bohannon and Smith 1987, Barnes and Johnson 2008).
- Consideration must be given to the practical application of these measurements where a client may have long-standing hypertonus, contractures in their joints and associated muscle atrophy.
- If someone has global brain damage then this is not going to change, it may be possible to manage its manifestations with medication and physiotherapy, but it is never going to resolve.
- Some of the objective tests that Barnes and Johnson (2008) describe consider how muscles react during gait; however, for many individuals with LD this is something that they have never done or no longer do.
- Measurements such as the Goldsmith Windswept Deformity Measure are more specifically aimed at the postural problems associated with LD (Goldsmith et al 1992).
- This can only measure accurately intact hip joints that have not subluxed or dislocated. The latter two can only be definitely diagnosed by radiological evidence.
- Scoliosis is something encountered in LD and the component of the wind-sweeping phenomenon that pertains to spinal scoliosis is not measured using the Goldsmith's measure.
- Objective measurement of scoliosis tends to only occur when surgical intervention is being decided on or if a client has been reviewed regularly in a specialist clinic.
- For individuals that develop a postural scoliosis it is a challenge for LD physiotherapists to accurately measure this or overall asymmetrical posture.
- Digital photographs or video footage can be taken to monitor changes over time.

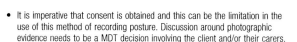

- It is imperative that consent is obtained and this can be the limitation in the use of this method of recording posture. Discussion around photographic evidence needs to be a MDT decision involving the client and/or their carers.

- Individuals with LD may also present with any acute or chronic condition that a member of the general population may have, e.g. rheumatology, orthopaedic or respiratory. Some more able individuals may be able to attend acute physiotherapy services, in general however most will be managed by their own LD physiotherapist.

- Assessment of such conditions will be the same in principle, but the physiotherapist assessing may have to modify their communication and handling skills to accommodate the individual's needs.

- Some of the objective measurements used to assess and treat may not be applicable, e.g. due to an individual's increased pain threshold, or the inability to distinguish between hot and cold or sharp and blunt, these may contraindicate the use of certain electrotherapy modalities.

- LD physiotherapists have to be inventive in how they gather information and treat the individual.

- The objective assessment of problems follows the same basic elements as the methods used for the assessment of the general population, however there may need to be some modification of the implementation of tests to enable the recording of information.

- When dealing with respiratory problems there may be occasions when an individual's asymmetrical posture may make auscultation a challenge. The trunk may be rotated or their ribs and the pelvis overlap, causing impingement of the lung and reducing functional respiration.

- Generally when physiotherapists perform suction they assume that their catheter will pass easily down to the lungs, with LD there may be associated anatomical abnormalities that make suction difficult to achieve.

- Fitness testing objective measures can be used such as grip strength, peak flow, and flexibility. However, patience and repetition may need to be applied, as individuals with LD may be anxious and agitated when faced with new experiences.

- Individuals with balance problems can be tested using the 'Tinetti Balance Scale' or the 'Get Up and Go Test'. These are used by physiotherapists working with clients in elderly care and dementia settings.

- There may need to be some modification but the core elements would be the same.

- A student or junior physiotherapist probably has all the objective assessment skills needed for working in LD, they just need to learn to be flexible and inventive in how they use them.

- When on placement or on rotation there will be more experienced physiotherapy staff that will be able to provide guidance during assessments.

- The physiotherapist may need to refresh their memories about how to use specific tools, but they will be able to demonstrate different ways of communicating and adapting the implementation of the tests.

- The objective measurements learnt during undergraduate training may or may not be useful in LD. If used some may not be sufficiently sensitive to monitor the small changes that LD individuals may undergo, e.g. the Physical Ability Scale (PAS) that has 7 levels evaluating sitting ability. PAS may be useful for gross movement evaluation, e.g. for LD clients that have had a stroke, but for more complex individuals the skills needed to show change from one level to another tend to be too great. Therefore monitoring sitting ability using this scale may show negligible change despite the individual improving in many areas.

- Outcome measures can be adapted to suit a specific clientele. For example, the Aquatic Therapy Association of Chartered Physiotherapists (ATACP) has promoted the use of an adaptation of Measured Yourself Medical Outcomes (MYMOP) (Paterson 1996).
- Within objective assessments goal setting is seen as an important part of the whole approach.
- If a patient with LD sustains a fracture, then the time scales for healing should be no different from the general population.
- However, for those LD clients with more complex problems their short- and long-term goals will vary greatly compared to patients without LD presenting with similar physical problems and being managed in the acute setting.

The references for this chapter can be found on www.expertconsult.com.

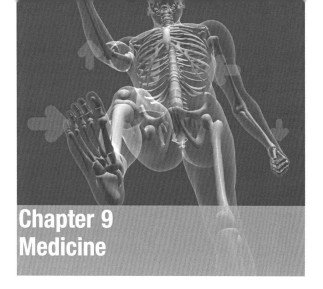

# Chapter 9
# Medicine

## Introduction

- The prospect of undertaking a medical placement or rotation within an acute hospital trust can fill a student or band 5 (newly qualified or not) with either a sense of trepidation or excitement.

- Medicine tends to be a placement or rotation that is not considered by many students or graduates to be 'desirable', unlike outpatients, ITU or paediatrics for example.

- What is involved in working in medicine tends to be poorly understood by both students and graduates alike.

- Medicine is a diverse speciality where physiotherapy can really make a difference to patients' independence and the overall quality of their lives.

- From a professional and developmental perspective medicine can provide an environment where fundamental knowledge and skills can be acquired which will be valuable and applicable to all other areas of physiotherapy practice, that are likely to be encountered throughout a professional career.

- The most likely location of a medical rotation is within an acute hospital trust, the size of which can be variable.

- It is realistic to say that a band 5 will be responsible for more than one medical ward, and students may also find that they have patients dispersed over a number of wards.

- Medical wards may encompass any number of beds from 20 upwards.

- There has been an increase in average age of the population in recent years and this poses increasing challenges for clinical staff working in the area of medicine when it comes to providing safe and effective management of their patients.

- There have been rising numbers of admissions and the associated demand for beds has often been accompanied by a reduction in the number of acute beds that are available as a result of efficiency cuts in budgets.
- Many of these changes have followed the introduction of government policies and it is these policies that have provided the drivers for the production of clinical guidelines (DOH 2010, NHS 2000, Reeves et al, 2003).
- The Department of Health white paper: 'Equity and Excellence: Liberating the NHS' (2010) outlines the future of the NHS, with Government recommendations suggesting reforms that are both challenging and far-reaching in terms of the cultural changes that they will bring about in the NHS (DOH 2010).
- The proposal is for the NHS to release up to £20 billion through efficiency savings, which will be reinvested to support improvements in quality of care, clinical outcomes and to provide a coherent, stable, enduring framework for quality and service improvement (DOH 2010).
- It is realistic to view the proposals as being the most significant and radical changes in the NHS in recent times that may change physiotherapy practice beyond recognition and will impact on the delivery of physiotherapy in the medicine setting (Dixon and Ham 2010).

## Conditions encountered in medicine

- All patients will be under the care of a consultant-led medical team for the duration of their admission in hospital.
- The conditions and pathologies that will be encountered within the speciality of medicine either as a presenting condition (PC) or past medical history (PMH) are diverse.
- It is not possible to cover these in depth in this volume, therefore a list of examples is provided to indicate the variety of conditions and experiences associated with medicine (Table 9.1).
- It is essential to have some knowledge of the condition a patient is presenting with and/or the patient's past medical history in order to perceive the patient holistically.

## The role of the physiotherapist and the multidisciplinary team (MDT)

- It is equally important to recognise the role of the physiotherapist during the patient's period of hospital admission.
- The process by which a patient is referred into the physiotherapy service will vary, depending on the system of preference within an individual hospital.
- Some units may operate a 'blanket referral' policy, where every patient on a particular ward has their physiotherapy needs assessed.
- Other organisations may operate a 'nurse-led' referral system, resulting in the nursing staff being able to refer patients to the ward physiotherapy service on an as-required basis.
- Some may follow the more historical system where only members of the consultant team are able to complete a referral, i.e. house officer (HO), senior house officer (SHO), registrar (Reg), senior registrar (Sen Reg) or the consultant themselves.

**Table 9.1** Specialist areas of practice and common conditions associated with medicine

| | |
|---|---|
| Cardiology | Acute coronary syndrome (ACS)<br>Angina<br>AF (atrial fibrillation)<br>MI (myocardial infarction)<br>CCF (congestive cardiac failure) |
| Respiratory | Chronic obstructive pulmonary disease (COPD)<br>Asthma<br>Emphysema<br>Pulmonary embolism<br>Tuberculosis (TB)<br>Upper or lower respiratory tract infections (URTI/LRTI)<br>Pleurisy<br>Hospital- or community-acquired pneumonia (HAP/CAP)<br>Bronchitis<br>Bronchiectasis |
| Neurology | Stroke<br>Head injuries<br>Multiple sclerosis<br>Parkinson's disease<br>Guillian–Barré<br>Transient ischaemic attack (TIA)<br>Dementia<br>Alzheimer's disease |
| Vascular | Peripheral vascular disease<br>Amputees<br>Intermittent claudication<br>Deep vein thrombosis (DVT) |
| Metabolic | Diabetes |
| Urinary | Urinary tract infections (UTI)<br>Kidney infections<br>Incontinence/behaviour change/acute confusion |
| Oncology | Any current or previous presentation/history of cancer |
| Cellulitis | Pain; decreased mobility/function; infection |
| Falls | Could be due to any of the above; decreased mobility or function; drug management |

- Alternatively a service may operate a mix and match of any of the above referral processes.
- MDT working is covered during the training of physiotherapy students in the university setting where it may seem to be a rather abstract concept in many instances.
- It is during placements or rotations that multiprofessional practice is placed into context.
- It is in clinical practice where MDT working can be seen to facilitate the efficient and effective management of patients, ensuring discharge from hospital occurs in the shortest possible time.

- During a medical placement/rotation the other members of the MDT that will come into contact with physiotherapists are; occupational therapists (OT), speech and language therapists (SALT), social workers (SW), dieticians, pharmacists, specialist nurses with an interest in chronic obstructive pulmonary disease, tissue viability, multiple sclerosis or Parkinson's disease.

- In the author's experience the use of a physiotherapy ward book can be an effective and informative method of keeping a record of the patients that have been referred into the service and can include specific information about when they have been seen or not and also highlight those that are deemed to be too ill for intervention.

- Ward books also offer an 'at a glance' view of the workload that includes the case mix, overall numbers of patients and levels of dependency.

- They can be found along with other medical records on the ward or in a designated physiotherapy area.

- Medical wards can be incredibly busy, therefore it is essential that ward physiotherapists remain aware of what patients are currently under their care, that they are confident when prioritising their workload, are clear about when patients were last seen and that they ensure timely intervention.

- If patients are not on the ward, as anticipated, the reason for this needs to be discovered, e.g. a patient may have been transferred to another ward or specialty, they may have been discharged or have self discharged or no longer require treatment, e.g. the patient has died.

## Prioritisation

- With the rising pressure to provide efficient services in health and social care the assessment and subsequent prioritisation of the patient care is imperative to ensure that they receive appropriate physiotherapy intervention in a timely and appropriate manner, according to their care needs and also in relation to their discharge plan.

- The workload tends to be much more variable on a medical ward than, for example, the predictable flow of patients every 20 or 30 minutes as experienced by physiotherapists in the outpatient setting.

- It is important to be able to manage time effectively in order that patients are appropriately assessed, that the physiotherapy interventions are defined for their particular needs and delivered in the appropriate time frame on any particular day.

- To be able to achieve this it is essential that the physiotherapist is able to prioritise their workload; if this is not done the patients will not be managed in the most efficient manner and will spend longer in hospital, further increasing pressure on beds.

- Prioritisation is a skill that needs to be developed.

- The physiotherapist needs to have an in-depth understanding of the presenting condition (PC), PMH and the associated risks of not seeing a patient within a desired time frame, if they are to manage their patients effectively and efficiently.

- In some organisations there may be a generic in-patient prioritisation document or process that will have been designed to assist physiotherapists in being able to identify high, medium and low priority, which is the equivalent of the 'must, should and could' process used in many musculoskeletal outpatient departments.

## Delegation

- Another important skill that physiotherapists need to become proficient at alongside of prioritisation is that of delegation.
- One of the most valuable members of the medical team is the physiotherapy assistant, who provides clinical support for the physiotherapist.
- They may assist the physiotherapist with patients that require the assistance of two or more staff to enable a treatment to be implemented safely and effectively.
- Assistants are also able to complete patient treatment inventions as directed by the physiotherapist, as long as they have been deemed to be confident and competent to do so and the task remains within the assistants' professional scope of practice.

## Seeking help

- It is important to highlight that if a student, or band 5 physiotherapist experiences difficulties with the management of their workload, or there is uncertainty about how to prioritise the patients on a daily basis, that these concerns are shared with a supervisor or more senior clinician working in the area.
- This is essential to ensure that patients receive the appropriate level of intervention and the advising clinician should be able to offer advice, help devise strategies about how to approach the work or propose joint working sessions to help build confidence and show the practical application of prioritising workload in the practice area.

## Assessment

- As with most physiotherapy assessments there are subjective and objective components to be completed.
- Patient information can be gathered from many sources on the wards, with medical, nursing and other professions, documentation being resources that can be accessed to assist the physiotherapist in the compilation of the subjective assessment, enabling a detailed picture to be developed of each patient referred for physiotherapy.
- In some hospitals multi-professional notes may be in operation, these are designed to reduce the amount of duplication of notes or repeated questioning of patients that may often occur.
- Before commencing a face-to-face assessment the physiotherapist will need to collect a significant amount of information.
- It is important to read and digest the pertinent issues from the medical notes, i.e. history of present condition (HPC)/past medical history (PMH)/drug history (DH)/social history (SH), and differential diagnosis.
- It is also useful to refer to information about medical investigations.
- The information from the notes will assist professional clinical reasoning and the physiotherapist to establish a clinical picture of each patient and their potential needs before a face-to-face meeting.
- Commonly encountered medical investigations, their findings and their relevance to physiotherapy assessment are covered in the following sections.

## Inflammatory markers

- On admission a patient may routinely have a full blood screen.
- An element of this investigation is looking at any changes in a patient's inflammatory markers (Table 9.2).

### C reactive protein (CRP) levels

- CRP is a plasma protein and increase in levels of this in the blood can be detected within 6 hours, with a final level being as much as 60 times normal levels.
- Raised levels of CRP are unequivocal evidence of inflammation (Randox website).
- Inflammation is the body's response to injury and the infection detected may be acute or chronic.

### Cardiac inflammatory markers

- From a cardiac perspective it is important to consider the specific blood tests that can be completed. When a patient is admitted to an accident and emergency department (A&E) or a step down equivalent with chest pain and a suspected myocardial infarction (MI) there are a number of investigations that may be carried out.
- Results from an ECG may be combined with results from blood tests and viewed in the context of the patient's presenting signs and symptoms and their PMH.
- An MI is major trauma to the cardiac muscle which will subsequently result in inflammation of the cardiac muscle to a varying degree depending on the severity of the infarction.
- This trauma and inflammation releases cardiac-specific enzymes, namely Troponin-T and Troponin-I.
- Troponin is a complex of three regular proteins that are integral to muscle contraction in skeletal and cardiac muscle but are not found in smooth muscle. The presence of troponin is used as an indicator for several heart disorders including MI. The subtypes Troponin-T and -I are specific indicators of damage to the myocardium.

| **Table 9.2** Inflammatory markers illustrating normal and clinically significant values | |
| --- | --- |
| White cell count (WCC) | Normal range: $4-11 \times 10^9$/L (4,000–11,000 per cubic millimetre of blood) |
| Erythrocyte sedimentation rate (ESR) | Normal range:<br>Men 12–19 mm/h<br>Women 18–23 mm/h<br>(within age range 20–90 years) |
| C reactive protein (CRP) | Normal level: 10 mg/L<br>Significant bacterial infection or acute inflammation: 40–200 mg/L<br>Serious bacterial infection: 300 mg/L or higher (Randox 2011) |

## Identifying the presence of infection

- When establishing if the cause of a patient's presenting condition is an infection, then investigating if any of their inflammatory markers are raised can confirm this as being one of the pieces of their clinical jigsaw puzzle.
- If one or all are raised this would suggest that a patient has an infection, the next step is to establish the cause.
- If considering a suspected respiratory infection a link could be made between the patient's signs and symptoms, arterial blood gas (ABGs) results, acid–base balance, X-ray findings and sputum sample results.
- Similarly if considering a urinary tract infection (UTI) the presenting signs and symptoms are important in the formation of a diagnosis in combination with urinalysis.

## Conclusion

- There is no one specific investigation or symptom that will be viewed as being definitive of a diagnosis in isolation.
- The whole picture of a patient's presentation will gradually come together following the completion of a full medical assessment.
- In many instances the information that a physiotherapist establishes during an assessment can further support and assist the medical teams with their ongoing treatment and management of individual patients and their presenting condition while the patient remains in hospital.

## Subjective assessment

- Although there is a certain amount of information that may have been extrapolated by the medical team or nursing staff there may be some additional physiotherapy-specific details that may need to be acquired from either the patient themselves or from their relatives and/or carers.
- Being in possession of an accurate social history is critical to physiotherapists assisting the patient with appropriate goal formulation and discharge planning.
- Social history (SH) relates to all the day-to-day aspects of independence, for example occupation present or previous, levels of indoor/outdoor mobility and endurance; aids required, washing and dressing, cooking, housework, hobbies, dependents, pets.
- Not only is it essential to document all the aspects of SH it is even more essential to be able to plot and identify changes within an individual's SH, especially if these changes can be correlated with episodes of illness, admissions to hospital or simply the natural progression of a long-term condition, e.g. COPD.
- A further vital piece of SH is identifying the type of accommodation that a patient has been admitted from. For example, has a patient been admitted from home, where they live independently and are normally able to manage stairs, or have they been admitted from a nursing home, where they require assistance with transfers, use a hoist and are only able to mobilise a few metres using a Zimmer frame and the assistance of two members of staff.
- It is important that the baseline of ability is identified as soon after admission as is possible.

- Another important consideration is the potential for the hospital environment to actually disable people.
- The author recalls a patient who was admitted with a UTI to an acute medical ward from their own home, where she lived independently.
- In hospital the bed was a different height to the patient's bed at home and the patient had not been admitted with her sliding board.
- This meant she was unable to transfer independently and mobilise in her wheelchair, which caused a great deal of frustration and the loss of dignity for that patient, who understandably was desperate to be discharged home simply in order to regain her independence.

- The process of discharge planning begins from the time of hospital admission and requires discussions to take place between health professionals on a regular and frequent basis to consider changes in the patient's condition and progression in respect of interventions.

- There are certain aspects of a patient's discharge that can be proactively planned for, e.g. if a patient has reported a long history of falls, then referral to a falls clinic can be organised along with support at home on discharge provided by an intermediate care team to include falls prevention training within the patient's own home.

- A patient with COPD can be referred to pulmonary rehabilitation or input from a COPD specialist nurse.

## Objective assessment

### Observation

- Observations include medical observations; blood pressure (BP); respiratory rate (RR); heart rate (HR); temperature, oxygen saturation ($SaO_2$); which are normally recorded by the nursing team and documented on the patient's observation chart and importantly what can be seen when the physiotherapist visits the patient.
- The following observations can be made:
- Is the patient alert?
- Are they talking to patients in neighbouring beds or to themselves?
- Are they breathing regularly or short of breath?
- Are they spontaneously moving in the chair or bed?
- What is their colour like? Pale; flushed?
- What is their posture in bed or in a chair?
- Are they wearing glasses and/or hearing aid?
- Do they appear aware of their environment/surroundings?
- Are there any walking aids nearby – NB need to check any aids belong to the patient they are next to.

### Consent

- There are fundamental components of an objective assessment that are applicable to patients on a medical ward, irrespective of the reason for admission to hospital.
- Prior to any form of patient assessment it is essential that consent is gained from the patient (CSP 2004).

- Patient consent, whether it is written or verbal, needs to be obtained prior to any element of assessment or treatment. It is prudent to record that this has occurred within professional documentation.
- Similarly it is imperative that the patient's consent is obtained prior to discussing any aspect of their assessment findings or care plan with a next of kin, relative or carer.

## Muscle strength

- Upper limb and lower limb muscle groups, using the Oxford Scale grading 0–5.
- Comparison of the patient's left side against their right.

## Joint range of movement

- To include any specific joints involved in their presentation and the functional joints in the upper and lower limb, i.e. hip, knee, shoulder and wrist comparing the right and left.

## Sensation

- Generic assessment of both sides of the body should note the intact areas and identify patchy sensation or specific areas where sensation changes have occurred.
- The findings may indicate where the patient's skin integrity may be at risk.

## Current mobility and functional level

- This needs to be benchmarked against the patient's pre-admission status.
- The assessment should include bed mobility; transfers; mobility indoors and outdoors.
- This may involve liaison with the OTs regarding personal activities of daily living (PADL) and domestic activities of daily living (DADL).

## Stairs assessment

- If the patient has stairs at home then this will need to be included in the assessment.
- It will need to be determined if the patient is able to ascend and descend stairs and also if they are safe to do so.
- The need for aids or the addition of stair rails or a supplementary banister will need to be considered.

## Current endurance and fitness level compared to preadmission status

- When synthesising this information the question needs to be asked whether the objective outcomes assessed reflect the condition of the patient when they were at home.
- Did these contribute to the problem or did they impact on each other, e.g. if a patient has decreased ROM in the knee joint and has decreased muscle strength could these be contributing factors in the patient's declining levels of mobility and the occurrence of falls at home?

## Speciality-specific objective assessments

- In addition to the generic components of the objective assessment highlighted above there are more specific assessments that will need to be completed, that depend on the reason for admission and/or the patient's past medical history.
- The two specific objective assessment approaches that are used in medicine tend to have a cardiorespiratory and neurological basis.

## Cardiorespiratory assessment

- Breathing pattern.
- Is there obvious accessory muscle contraction?
- Is the patient demonstrating increased work of breathing?
- Is it possible to observe pursed lip breathing?
- Does the patient demonstrate shortness of breath at rest?
- Palpation
- Is the chest expanding equally on both sides?
- Can sputum crackles be felt?
- Auscultation
- Identification of abnormal breath sounds and/or added sounds
- Are breath sounds audible throughout the lung fields?
- Are the breath sounds normal, abnormal or diminished (Hough 2001)?
- Are there added sounds?
- Can crackles be heard? That could indicate the presence of unwanted secretions
- When are the crackles heard? early, mid or late inspiration?
- Are inspiratory or expiratory wheezes present?
- Expiratory wheeze with a prolonged period of expiration can be caused by bronchospasm, whereas an inspiratory and expiratory wheeze can occur as the result of there being an obstruction in the airways
- Pleural rub may occur when the patient has pleurisy, which is an inflammation of the pleural surface
- Pleural rub can sound like crunching on snow and is best auscultated over the lower lung fields (Hough 2001).
- Sputum or increased levels of secretions
- Colour and consistency.
- Mucus or pulmonary oedema
- Is there blood present indicating haemoptysis? And does this link with any PMH or with the current diagnosis?

## Investigations to aid assessment

- Sputum specimen analysis will assist in the identification of the pathogen responsible for the infection (Hough 2001).
- Chest X-ray (CXR) can identify issues such as fluid levels or consolidation of specific areas of the lungs.

- Bloods samples can indicate the presence of underlying pathology, e.g. inflammatory markers.
- Arterial blood gases (ABGs)

Normal values:
  $PaO_2$: 11–14 kPa (80–100 mmHg)
  $SaO_2$: 95–98%
  $PaCO_2$: 4.7–6.0 kPa (35–45 mmHg)
Acid–base balance:
  pH: 7.35–7.45
$HCO_3$ (bicarbonate levels):
  normal 22–26 mmol/L
Metabolic acidosis:
  <22 mmol/L
Metabolic alkalosis:
  >26 mmol/L
Base excess
  Normal: minus 2 to plus 2 mmol/L
  Metabolic acidosis: <–2 mmol/L
  Metabolic alkalosis: >2 mmol/L (Hough, 2001).

## Neurological assessment

- Assessment will include the following areas:
- Movement which will pay particular attention to the quality of movement
- Tone
- Rigidity
- Sensation
- Co-ordination
- Proprioception
- Neglect
- Communication
- Postural assessment.
- The assessment of swallowing and speech is not within a physiotherapist's scope of practice.
- However, if a physiotherapist has concerns or is aware that a patient is having difficulties managing their secretions and therefore may be at risk of aspirating then it is essential that the respiratory status is assessed and regularly reviewed.
- With regards to communication a physiotherapist can liaise with the SALT team for specific intervention to improve the patient's ability to communicate.

The references for this chapter can be found on www.expertconsult.com.

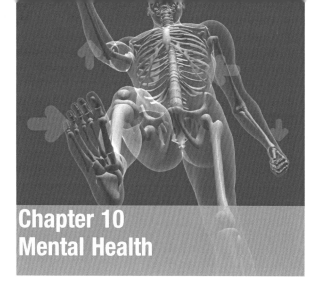

# Chapter 10
# Mental Health

## Introduction

### What is the role of the physiotherapist in mental health?

- This is always the first question a physiotherapist working in mental health will be asked and often by other physiotherapists.

- It is quite simply physiotherapy, as defined by the Chartered Society of Physiotherapy (CSP), (www.csp.org.uk): a profession that:

  *uses physical approaches to promote, maintain and restore physical, psychological and social well-being, …*

- In mental health the psychological disorder may be the primary health risk and physiotherapeutic skills may be used to reduce this, but it may also be the case that on assessment it is physical dysfunction and the treatment of this that is of paramount importance in the holistic management of the person.

- In all cases it is important to assess and treat the physical difficulties and dysfunction alongside any psychological dysfunction that may be present.

- Working with the multidisciplinary team (MDT) is essential, as it is in many specialties of physiotherapy. In the field of mental health the difference may be that the physiotherapist is regarded as the physical expert in the team.

- The physiotherapist's knowledge has to be broad, so that it is possible to assess a wide range of conditions and evaluate which are appropriate for mental health physiotherapy intervention and which need another specialist physiotherapist, c.g. musculoskeletal.

## Concerns of students and clinicians without experience in mental health

- Research undertaken at Cardiff University with students prior to beginning mental health placements has shown that pre placement education helps the student (Sarin 2008). This should be no surprise; however the main reported advantage was not to do with physiotherapy assessment, but rather assuaging the student's fear of violence and psychological trauma.

- Challenging behaviour management should be addressed within any team working in a mental health setting. It is the responsibility of the individual to ask for training if it is not offered. On in-patient wards, staff are likely to wear alarms in order to summon help for patients or colleagues. In the community, safeguards will include: having clear lone working policies and procedures, which in most cases insist that students or junior staff always work with an experienced member of the team (www.hse.gov.uk).

- As in any health setting the safety of the patient/client and staff is of paramount importance and risk assessment of the treatment environment and of the individual client should be undertaken in all circumstances, in relation to all aspects of safety. Knowledge of the patient is essential and awareness of family and physical environment factors will increase your confidence in working with this client group.

## Patients

- A physiotherapist working in mental health will encounter patients with musculoskeletal, neurological, respiratory and other physical dysfunction who also have psychological difficulties or who are experiencing psychological aspects of disease or disorder (Everett et al 2003).

- The type of patients that will be encountered will depend greatly on the structure of the service in which the physiotherapist is working.

- It may vary from primary care for mild to moderate depression and anxiety to long-term and enduring illness in supported housing or may be an acute adult in-patient service or a specialist dementia service.

- The term used for people accessing mental health care is often 'service user', sometimes 'client' and rarely 'customer'.

- Working with older adults however the term 'patient' is most often used.

- Service user, patient and client will all be used in this chapter and the case studies included as part of the web resource accompanying this book.

- Patients are divided by age groups and conditions as follows:
- Adults of working age
a  Acute disorder
b  Long-term and enduring mental health
- Older adults
a  Anxiety, depression
b. Dementia
- Child and adolescent
- and also by care groups as follows:
a  Eating disorder
b  Conversion disorder

c  Substance misuse

d  Forensic services.

## The physiotherapy setting

- Experience will vary throughout the UK, with some mental health services there is discrete physiotherapy input in primary, secondary or tertiary services.

- For other patients, seen by their GP or primary care psychological service they may receive their physiotherapy from a general outpatient department.

- Adults referred to a Community Mental Health Team (CMHT), are most likely to be seen by a general physiotherapist initially.

- If patients are referred to a mental health physiotherapist it is usually because of the rigid structure of the process in a general outpatient department, such as the standards relating to appointment times, the discharge of patients if they 'do not attend', fast turnaround assessment and treatment times, often precluding a successful outcome for patients with psychological disorders (Griffiths 2009).

## Knowledge specific to mental health

### What is mental health?

- A useful definition of mental health is that used by the World Health Organization (WHO):

  *Mental health is a state of well-being in which the individual realizes his or her own abilities, can cope with the normal stresses of life, can work productively and fruitfully and is able to make a contribution to his or her community (WHO 2010).*

- The Mental Health Foundation has defined a mentally healthy individual as one who can:
- Develop emotionally, creatively, intellectually and spiritually
- Initiate, develop and sustain mutually satisfying personal relationships
- Face problems, resolve them and learn from them
- Be confident and assertive
- Be aware of others and empathise with them
- Use and enjoy solitude
- Play and have fun
- Laugh, both at themselves and at the world (http://www.mentalhealth.org.uk/welcome/).

### What is mental disorder?

- Defining mental disorder is difficult, because it is not one condition, but a group of conditions.

- There is intense debate about which conditions are or should be included in the definition of mental disorders.

- Specifically in the UK, in relation to personality disorder and substance misuse and for some eating disorders there is disagreement as to their classification.

- For legal purposes, the UK's Mental Health Act (2007) defines mental disorder succinctly as, 'any disorder or disability of the mind'. It is clear that there is a marked circularity to this statement as the WHO states that mental disorder is more than the absence of mental health.

- The focus in this chapter will be on those disorders which are recognised and treated within the NHS and which are likely to be presented to a community mental health trust (CMHT) or mental health inpatient setting.

- It should be remembered that there are many disorders which the physiotherapist may encounter in any physical medical specialty and in general outpatient departments and so this information should be applicable to any physiotherapy setting.

## Diagnostic systems

- Both the WHO, International Classification of Diseases, 10th edition (ICD10) and American Psychiatric Association Diagnostic and Statistical Manual-IV (DSM IV) are used to diagnose mental disorder.

- Their purpose is to make a diagnosis and this is not always appropriate as many of the disorders are not necessarily a disease in the medical sense.

- Mental disorder may be described in a biological system focusing on changes in brain chemistry, e.g. hormones, genetic formation.

- Psychological systems focus on personal development and thinking, e.g. cognition. Social systems focus on environment, social structures and family relationship.

- A mental disorder may be described using any individual or combination of these systems.

- The main categories of ICD10 are:
- Organic disorders, e.g. dementia
- Pyschotic disorders, e.g. schizophrenia and delusional disorders
- Mood disorders, e.g. depression and mania
- Neurotic disorders, e.g. panic, anxiety, obsessive compulsive disorder.
- Physiological disturbances and physical-based syndromes, e.g. eating disorders (WHO 2010).

## Disorders commonly encountered by physiotherapists

- The following descriptions and symptom lists are drawn from WHO ICD10.
- Also included are some definitions from the support organisation 'MIND', which give a more person-centred description of mental disorders.
- It should be noted that there is still discussion about what schizophrenia is and the MIND website provides information relating to current thinking about schizophrenia (Henriques 2011).

### Depression

- Depression is a common mental disorder that presents with depressed mood, loss of interest or pleasure, feelings of guilt or low self-worth, disturbed sleep or appetite, low energy, and poor concentration.

- These problems can become chronic or recurrent and lead to substantial impairments in an individual's ability to take care of his or her everyday responsibilities.

- At its worst, depression can lead to suicide, a tragic fatality associated with the loss of about 850 000 lives every year (WHO 2010).
- To come to a diagnosis of depression the symptoms should be present for at least 2 weeks and include four of the symptoms below plus at least one additional symptom:
- Depressed mood to a degree that is definitely abnormal for the individual, should be present for most of the day and almost every day, largely uninfluenced by circumstances, and sustained for at least 2 weeks
- Loss of interest or pleasure in activities that are normally pleasurable
- Decreased energy or increased fatigability
- Loss of confidence and self-esteem
- Unreasonable feelings of self-reproach or excessive and inappropriate guilt
- Recurrent thoughts of death or suicide, or any suicidal behaviour
- Complaints or evidence of diminished ability to think or concentrate, such as indecisiveness or vacillation
- Change in psychomotor activity, with agitation or retardation
- Sleep disturbance of any type.

## Bipolar disorder

- Bipolar disorder has in the past been termed 'manic depression', which gives some idea of the presentation.
- It is a mood disorder which has many combinations of low and high mood with or without psychotic symptoms.

## Schizophrenia

- Schizophrenia is a severe form of mental illness affecting about 7 per thousand of the adult population, mostly in the age group 15–35 years.
- Although the incidence is low (3 in every 10,000), the prevalence is high due to chronicity (WHO 2010).
- It can be described as a psychosis.
- The view is that a person cannot distinguish their own intense thoughts, ideas, perceptions and imaginings from reality.
- A person might be hearing voices, or may believe that other people can read their mind and control their thoughts.
- There is a view that these symptoms are logical or natural reactions to adverse life events. There is a need to think about individual experience, and the importance of understanding what the experiences mean to the individual.
- Hearing voices, holds a different significance within different cultures and spiritual belief systems (MIND 2010).
- There are many subdivisions of the definition which can be found on the WHO website but all have in common the symptoms stated above often both positive and negative symptoms.
- For some patients though, negative symptoms predominate. These symptoms characterise simple schizophrenia.
- This has a slow progressive development over a period of at least 1 year, of all three of the following:

- A significant and consistent change in the overall quality of some aspects of personal behaviour, manifest as loss of drive and interests, aimlessness, idleness, a self-absorbed attitude, and social withdrawal.
- Gradual appearance and deepening of 'negative' symptoms such as marked apathy, paucity of speech, underactivity, blunting of affect, passivity and lack of initiative, and poor non-verbal communication (by facial expression, eye contact, voice modulation and posture).
- Marked decline in social, scholastic, or occupational performance.

## Dementia

- Dementia is not one disease, but rather a group of diseases that lead slowly to memory loss and confusion, affecting people's personality and behaviour.
- There is a decline in ability to carry out normal, everyday activities (MIND 2010).
- The most common types of dementia are vascular, Alzheimer's and Lewy body, but there are also dementias that are caused by alcohol use, syphilis and other disease processes.

## Medications which might impact on physiotherapy intervention

### Medication for schizophrenia

- Antipsychotic medications are used to treat schizophrenia and schizophrenia-related disorders.
- Some of these medications have been available since the mid-1950s.
- They are also called conventional 'typical' antipsychotics, e.g. chlorpromazine (Thorazine or Largactil) and haloperidol (Haldol).
- In the 1990s, new antipsychotic medications were developed, called second-generation, or 'atypical' antipsychotics.
- Atypical antipsychotics include:
- Risperidone (Risperdal)
- Olanzapine (Zyprexa)
- Quetiapine (Seroquel)
- Ziprasidone (Geodon)
- Aripiprazole (Abilify).
- Side effects of many antipsychotics include:
- Drowsiness
- Dizziness when changing positions
- Blurred vision
- Rapid heartbeat
- Sensitivity to the sun
- Skin rashes
- Menstrual problems for women
- Agranulocytosis, which is a loss of the white blood cells that help a person fight infection. Patients taking clozapine must get their white blood cell counts checked regularly.
- Typical antipsychotic side effects include:
- Rigidity
- Persistent muscle spasms

- Tremors
- Restlessness.
- Long-term use may lead to tardive dyskinesia (TD). TD causes muscle movements a person can't control, commonly around the mouth. TD can range from mild to severe. Sometimes TD can cease or partially recover after stopping the medication.
- Atypical anti-psychotic side effects include:
- Major weight gain and changes in a person's metabolism
- Increased risk of diabetes and high cholesterol levels.
- A person's weight, glucose levels, and lipid levels should be monitored regularly by a doctor while taking an atypical antipsychotic medication.

## Medication for depression

- Depression is commonly treated with antidepressant medications.
- Antidepressants work to balance neurotransmitters such as serotonin, norepinephrine (noradrenaline), and dopamine in order to affect mood and emotional responses.
- The most popular types of antidepressants are called selective serotonin reuptake inhibitors (SSRIs).
- These include:
- Fluoxetine (Prozac)
- Citalopram (Celexa)
- Sertraline (Zoloft)
- Paroxetine (Paxil).
- Other types of antidepressants are serotonin and norepinephrine re-uptake inhibitors (SNRIs).
- SNRIs are similar to SSRIs and include venlafaxine (Effexor) and duloxetine (Cymbalta).
- SSRIs and SNRIs cause fewer side effects than the older classes of antidepressants.
- Antidepressants may cause mild side effects that usually do not last long.
- The most common side effects associated with SSRIs and SNRIs include:
- Headache, which usually goes away within a few days.
- Nausea, which usually goes away within a few days.
- Sleeplessness or drowsiness, which may happen during the first few weeks but then goes away.
- Agitation.
- Tricyclic antidepressants which have been replaced in most cases by SNRIs and SSRIs can cause the following side effects:
- Dry mouth
- Constipation
- Bladder problems
- Sexual problems
- Blurred vision
- Drowsiness.

- Patients taking monoamine oxidase inhibitors (MAOIs; late-stage antidepressants) need to pay attention to dietary intake as these can interact with certain constituents of foods (tyramine) and predispose the individual to increased blood pressure and stroke.

## Medications for bipolar disorder

- Bipolar disorder is commonly treated with mood stabilisers.
- Sometimes, antipsychotics and antidepressants are used along with a mood stabiliser.
- Lithium is a very effective mood stabiliser.
- Anticonvulsant medications also are used as mood stabilisers, e.g. valproic acid.
- Atypical antipsychotic medications are sometimes used to treat symptoms of bipolar disorder, often in conjunction with other medications.

## Medication for anxiety disorder

- Antidepressants, anti-anxiety medications, and beta-blockers are the most common medications used for anxiety disorders.
- SSRIs such as fluoxetine (Prozac), sertraline (Zoloft), escitalopram (Lexapro), paroxetine (Paxil), and citalopram (Celexa) are commonly prescribed for panic disorder, OCD, PTSD, and social phobia.
- The SNRI venlafaxine (Effexor) is commonly used to treat generalised anxiety disorder (GAD).
- Some tricyclic antidepressants work well for anxiety, e.g. imipramine (Tofranil), is prescribed for panic disorder and GAD and clomipramine (Anafranil) is used to treat OCD.
- The anti-anxiety medications called benzodiazepines can start working more quickly than antidepressants, e.g. clonazepam (Klonopin), which is used for social phobia and GAD, lorazepam (Ativan), which is used for panic disorder and alprazolam (Xanax), which is used for panic disorder and GAD.
- Beta-blockers control some of the physical symptoms of anxiety, such as trembling and sweating, e.g. propranolol (Inderal) is a beta-blocker used to treat heart conditions and high blood pressure.
- Common side effects for benzodiazepines are drowsiness and dizziness.
- Other possible side effects of beta-blockers include: fatigue, cold hands, dizziness, weakness and a worsening of asthma and diabetes, if present.

## Physiotherapy assessment

- Assessment aspects for adults with acute mental illness, older adults with dementia, adults with long-term and enduring mental illness will be considered.
- It is the attitude, choice of appropriate approach and consideration of the physiotherapist that can have the biggest impact on the assessment.
- Eating disorder, child and adolescent mental health and substance misuse are not covered in this volume, suggested reading is included in the online material.

### Types of referral

- In acute adult wards the most often received referrals are for pain in neck, back, limb joints plus assessment for exclusion of a physical cause for a behaviour, e.g. falling, shaking.

- In older adult wards referrals may also be for above conditions, but mobility is the main concern.
- Co-morbidities of stroke, Parkinson's/parkinsonism, diabetes and epilepsy may all exist alongside the primary diagnoses of functional or organic mental health disorders.

## Assessment process

- This will be similar to the assessment undertaken in other areas of physiotherapy.
- In mental health the specialist skills required are in communication, flexibility of approach, and the ability to work with patients.
- Physiotherapy assessment will form a component part of a MDT assessment.
- Knowledge of the symptoms and medication in mental disorder, how these might affect the patient's ability to function and comply with planned treatment is essential.

### Subjective information

- Physiotherapy records should encapsulate all relevant medical, psychological and pharmacological information.
- The psychological disorder may be the main focus of the rest of the team, therefore referrals may be lacking in detail or factual content about medical aspects of the patient's history.
- Patient's records will give, in most cases, a diagnosis, medication list and social background.
- Patient records are gradually moving towards being stored electronically, which has the advantage that they will be available and legible when they need to be accessed.
- Mental health patients may have a care programme approach (CPA), which as the name suggests should be a record of the service users' needs and the processes by which those needs will be met.
- Patients who have more than six interventions from a psychiatric professional or who are seen by more than one professional should have a CPA, which will be overseen by a care co-ordinator.
- The care co-ordinator may be a community psychiatric nurse (CPN), a doctor, an occupational therapist or a social worker and in some organisations a physiotherapist will take on this role.
- If a physiotherapist is the care co-ordinator it is usually because of specific physical health needs of the patient, or due to the specific skills set of the therapist.
- Information gained from the service user can vary from being clear and precise to confused and muddled or even imaginary, for those with psychosis or dementia.
- A large part of the skill in assessment approach is differentiation of factual information.
- However there must be respect for the patient and their view of the history of their illness.
- Information about both the psychological illness and physical disorder, must inform an assessment.

- Cultural and ethnic requirements of the patient need to be considered. This should be checked prior to assessment and discussed as part of the consent process.

## Assessment of adults of working age with a musculoskeletal condition

### Case example: Lower limb fracture, in-patient setting, acute episode of psychosis

- A lower limb fracture is a common referral for young males and may be related to:
- Trauma, fall, RTA
- Self harm/attempted suicide by jumping from height
- Outcome of fleeing from perceived threats, i.e. paranoid thoughts of persecution
- Assault.
- The cause may not be clear from the referral, so research into the background is essential.
- If the service user is in an acute state of psychosis then questioning is likely to be inappropriate.
- However, it may be possible to assess by observation, e.g. the ease of movement with walking aids and the condition of the leg above and below a plaster.
- Perception of pain in people with psychosis or mood disorders may be distorted in either direction, from hypersensitive to no experience of pain, where pain would be expected.
- Assessment of pain can involve the use of a visual analogue scale (VAS) if the service user is able, but this may have to be defined through observation.
- Non verbal expression of pain may be by facial expression, repeated touching of the affected part, excessive laughing or agitation.
- Discussion with the MDT regarding pain management should be part of treatment plan.
- If the service user is receiving antipsychotic medication, e.g. olanzapine they may be experiencing side effects such as drowsiness or dizziness when changing positions, blurred vision or a rapid heartbeat, all of which could affect their ability to comply with assessment and this should be taken into consideration.
- It will be the physiotherapist who has to provide the patient with information about post operative protocols and also translate orthopaedic reports from medical jargon into lay terms that can be understood by the patient, e.g. NWB, non weight bearing, PWB partial weight bearing and to explain which bone is damaged and what the healing process may be.
- Knowledge of healing times and weight-bearing protocols is essential.
- Liaising with other teams and communication of information to the MDT, and the service user if appropriate, are key physiotherapy skills.
- The risk of complications, e.g. deep vein thrombosis may not have been judged as high by the trauma team as they see the service user as young and active with the only risk factor being a lower limb cast.
- However, if the service user is in an isolative or paranoid phase they may be very immobile and may not take advice.

- The potential risk factors should be part of the physiotherapy assessment and findings must be shared with the MDT.
- A patient might not be able to understand the process of crutch walking, due to their level of psychosis or of general understanding.
- The physiotherapist must be able to assess this and share the findings with the MDT.
- Measurements of range of movement of the hip and knee, if a below knee cast is present or just hip, if the patient is in an above knee cast, should be taken.
- Upper limb strength and range of movement of the joints should be recorded.
- Where possible these should be checked using hands on assessment; however, with a psychotic patient this may not be possible as consent may not be given. In this instance observation will be the closest method of achieving an objective measurement.
- Occupational tasks can be used to assess range and to some extent strength; this is a good technique to develop, e.g. getting the person to reach up to get something for you or for themselves, or simply taking and passing back a reasonably heavy object.
- Personal safety on the ward is a consideration which will need to be assessed along with the rest of the MDT.
- It may be unsafe to give a patient with acute illness a pair of crutches.
- The risks are manifold and may include another patient who does not understand the consequences of pulling crutches away or, who without any malice, might push the person with crutches just to see what happens. The crutches could also end up being used as a weapon, either by the user or another patient.
- There are potential concerns when the patient is on an intensive care ward, where acute illness and the accompanying impulsive behaviour can be hazardous to the patient and other people in the ward.
- Where a patient may have a history of violence to themselves or others, e.g. in a forensic unit the physiotherapist may need to decide upon an alternative to crutches such as a wheelchair.

**Adult referred for general fitness/weight management for acute depression**
- Persons with long-term and enduring mental disorder are much more likely to have poor general health (MacDonald and O'Hara 1998, Tudor 1996).
- General well being is part of the remit of the physiotherapist in mental health (Everett et al 2003).
- Physiotherapy teams may include technical instructors (TI) or sports instructors.
- A patient referred for improvement of fitness may be assessed by the TI using a health screening tool and only if specific physical problems are found would the referral move to the physiotherapist.
- A pathway for this is covered in the treatment volume.
- A junior physiotherapist may be responsible for managing this process.
- Alongside physical screening psychological tests such as Beck Anxiety Inventory (BAI) or the Hospital Anxiety and Depression Scale (HADS) are used to give some indication of the baseline levels of anxiety and depression of the patient.

- Weight can be measured if a patient, wishes; weight management may include the use of BMI, waist circumference, activity level, plus questions about diet, smoking, and alcohol use in an assessment.

**Older adult with dementia, referred as a falls risk**

- Assessments for older adults will undoubtedly centre on general mobility and falls risk.
- The nursing team may have carried out a falls risk assessment on admission highlighting the need for physiotherapy intervention or it may be the physiotherapist that undertakes all falls risk assessments.
- There are a number of tools for assessing the risk of falls.
- Organisations may adapt tools to suit the requirements of their service. Examples of falls assessment tools include;
- STRATIFY (Oliver et al 1997)
- FRAT, Falls Risk Assessment Tool
- FULBROOK Local assessment containing triggers
- Assessment should evaluate mobility, strength, balance and confidence.
- The Elderly Mobility Scale (EMS) can be adapted for use in patients with dementia with the useful elements being sit to stand, and timed walk and movement to and from lying.
- Confidence or fear of falling can be assessed using a VAS.
- A simple facial expression indicator is an alternative where the patient chooses the picture of the facial expression which best represents their feelings about walking.
- In assessing older adults in the earlier stages of dementia the following elements are key; communication, patience, expectation of success (Oddy 2003, 2011).
- Consider communication in three areas:
- Giving
- Receiving
- Response.
- In the early stages of dementia short-term memory loss and confusion may be present.
- The other limiting factor for assessment will be the ability of the patient to process instructions or requests.
- Therefore questioning should include; clear, single subject questions and simple directions.
- It is important to allow time for the patient to process the instruction and to respond either verbally or physically.
- Advice points
- Approach the patient from the front
- Respect their personal space
- Address the patient by their name and make eye contact
- Keep body movements smooth and unhurried
- Speak clearly in a manner acceptable to an adult
- Be courteous
- Use appropriate facial expressions.

- It is also useful to use familiar or local expressions and base your requests on goals, e.g. walk to the bathroom.
- As with all communication techniques some will work better than others for different people.
- The stage of dementia will affect the success of communication styles.
- An empathetic and reassuring approach delivered in an adequate time frame will ensure an assessment occurs which identifies risk elements and enables the production of a plan to improve the safe mobility of the patient.

It is important to remember that patients with mental health disorders will be encountered in any area of physiotherapy practice.

Wherever the patient is encountered the physiotherapy skills can be applied through good communication, risk assessment and innovation to improve both the physical and psychological health and well being of each patient.

The references for this chapter can be found on www.expertconsult.com.

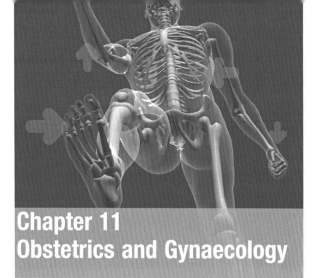

# Chapter 11
# Obstetrics and Gynaecology

## The role of the women's health physiotherapist

- Physiotherapy has been involved in obstetric care since the early 1900s due to the ground-breaking work of Minnie Randell at St Thomas' Hospital, London (Moscucci 2003).
- The formation of the Obstetric Physiotherapy Association in 1948 made it one of the first physiotherapy clinical interest groups.
- Obstetric physiotherapists expanded their role to encompass gynaecology, with the clinical interest group reflecting this in the title Association of Chartered Physiotherapists in Obstetrics and Gynaecology (ACPOG) in 1976.
- As physiotherapy has developed during the last 40 years, so has the management of women's health and in 1994 the association was renamed as the Association of Chartered Physiotherapists in Women's Health (ACPWH), to recognise the work done for women's health in general.
- This, however, does not reflect the volume of work carried out by many women's health (WH) physiotherapists treating male incontinence and erectile dysfunction.
- With 700 members worldwide the association is also a founder member of the International Organization of Physical Therapists in Women's Health (IOPTWH).
- WH physiotherapists are involved in the 4 spheres of physiotherapy; health promotion, prevention, treatment and rehabilitation, as defined by the World Confederation for Physical Therapy (WCPT 1999).
- This may involve promoting healthy lifestyles and posture in pregnancy or preventing pelvic floor dysfunction through teaching normal bladder and bowel function; treating musculoskeletal dysfunctions occurring in pregnancy or urinary incontinence as the consequence of pelvic floor dysfunction. These problems require the WH physiotherapist to draw on core skills of rehabilitation in order to improve or resolve a patient's problems.

- Physiotherapy departments which provide women's health services vary in the breadth of care they offer.
- The following list outlines services that WH physiotherapists may be involved in:
- Health promotion classes In pregnancy
- Back or pelvic girdle pain classes
- Parent education classes
- Antenatal exercise classes
- Aquanatal classes
- Treatment of musculoskeletal problems during pregnancy and post birth
- Postnatal exercise classes
- Inpatient obstetric care
- Inpatient gynaecology care
- In- and outpatient breast care
- Treatment of pelvic floor dysfunction in men and women
- Lymphoedema services.

## Obstetrics

When first entering a WH setting there will be terminology and processes that a student or physiotherapist may not have encountered previously. For example, the term 'gravida' describes the number of times a woman has conceived a pregnancy, and 'parity' describes the number of times a women has delivered a viable baby (classified as >24 weeks).

### Physiotherapy services in obstetrics

- Treatment of musculoskeletal changes in pregnancy and puerperium.
- Back care classes in pregnancy.
- Antenatal exercise classes.
- Postnatal exercise classes.
- Parent education classes.
- Ward based education and treatment pre- and post-delivery.

## Physiological changes in pregnant women

- The physiological changes that occur through pregnancy place increasing demands on a woman's body, which should not be underestimated (Mantle et al 2004).
- Pregnant women are often not aware of the rapid changes that occur to their body and may present with symptoms that concern them greatly.
- WH physiotherapists have the ability to inform and educate pregnant women about the normal physiological changes that occur during this period and in turn reduce their anxiety.
- Physiotherapists can also identify neuromusculoskeletal changes, treat and manage dysfunctions with their knowledge of the body.
- It is therefore important that physiotherapists working in obstetrics fully understand the normal physiological and musculoskeletal changes in pregnancy in order to identify possible abnormalities.

- The following sections discuss some of the more common physiological and musculoskeletal changes in pregnancy, however this is not inclusive.
- The changes during pregnancy can be broadly split into:
- Hormonal changes and their consequences
- Cardiovascular system changes
- Changes associated with the growth of the fetus
- Musculoskeletal adaptations in response to mother's increase in body weight.

## Hormonal changes and their consequences

- There remains a lot to learn about the hormonal changes in pregnancy and importantly for the physiotherapist their role as a causative factor of musculoskeletal pain.
- It seems that progesterone, oestrogen and relaxin have an important role in some of the physiological and anatomical changes in pregnancy.
- All three are produced by the corpus luteum up to 10 weeks of gestation, when the placenta also starts to produce them and fully takes over this role from the second trimester onwards (12 weeks).
- Relaxin is thought to peak in the first trimester and then drops by 20% to remain steady for the remaining trimesters.

### Effects of progesterone

- Reduction in tone of smooth muscle, resulting in:
- Reduced peristaltic movement, so food may stay longer in the stomach, coupled with an increase of water absorption in the colon leads to constipation.
- Slower bladder emptying.
- Dilatation of the ureters and lengthening to accommodate size of the fetus.
- Urethral tone is reduced, which may result in stress incontinence.
- Reduced tone in the smooth muscles of the blood vessels, leading to varicose veins and hot hands due to pooling of fluid.
- Increase in nasal and vaginal production.
- Increase in temperature by 0.5–1.0°C. Pregnant women often feel warm and the temperature of the treatment area needs to considered, so they do not feel uncomfortably warm.
- Reduction in alveolar and arterial $pCO_2$ tension.
- Pregnant women will be increasingly short of breath, even at low levels of exercise, which may lead to hyperventilation.
- Development of the alveolar and glandular milk-producing cells in the breasts. Breast size enlarges from early on in pregnancy which can change posture and cause strain to the thoracic or cervical spine.
- Increased storage of fat.

### Effects of oestrogens

- Increase in growth of uterus and breast ducts.
- Increasing levels of prolactin to prepare breasts for lactation.
- May prime receptor sites for relaxin.
- Increase in water retention.
- Increase in vaginal glycogen, predisposing to thrush.

## Effects of relaxin

- Gradual replacement of collagen with a remodelled modified form that has greater extensibility and pliability.

- Inhibition of myometrial activity during pregnancy up to 28 weeks, after which women can then become aware of Braxton Hicks contractions.

- Uterus distends from its usual 'small pear' size holding 6 ml of fluid to its full-term size of holding 5000 ml of fluid.

- There is controversy surrounding the role of relaxin as a cause of musculoskeletal pain. Since being discovered in 1926, relaxin has traditionally been thought to be the main reason for musculoskeletal pain in pregnancy.

- It has been presumed that manual therapy is not beneficial for joints that are in effect hypermobile.

- However, recent research has found that there is no correlation between serum levels of relaxin and pain.

- There is also no evidence to confirm that those with increased joint laxity or stiffness have an increased incidence of pain.

- It is now generally considered that relaxin is a causal factor in musculoskeletal pain in pregnancy; however pain is not caused by general increase in mobility, rather an asymmetrical difference between joints, particularly the sacroiliac joints.

## Cardiovascular system changes

- Blood volume increases by 40% to supply the increasing demands of the uterus and placenta.

- This is not accompanied by an increase in red blood cells, only plasma, so the haemoglobin levels fall to around 80%. This is known as physiological anaemia, which may result in tiredness and malaise.

- The heart increases in size and accommodates more blood, so the stroke volume rises and the cardiac output increases by 30–50%. Exercise will produce an increase in cardiac output, therefore this should be considered when teaching an exercise programme to a pregnant woman.

- Later in pregnancy, the weight of the fetus may compress the aorta and vena cava in the supine position causing dizziness and in extreme circumstances unconsciousness. This is known as supine hypotension. Not all women will suffer from this condition, however. Physiotherapists need to be aware about the potential effects of supine lying later on in pregnancy.

- Prolonged vigorous exercise should be avoided as this will result in redistribution of the cardiac output to the working muscles and away from the abdominal organs, importantly the uterus and placenta (Artal et al 1991).

## Changes associated with the growth of the fetus

### Respiratory system

- The growth of the fetus causes changes to the respiratory system by displacing the diaphragm upwards by 4 cm or more.

- This causes the ribs to flare outwards and the subcostal angle to increase from 68° to 103° and can cause breathlessness, as the respiratory excursion is limited at the lung bases.

- The costochondral junctions may become more hypermobile and therefore costal margin pain or rib ache is not uncommon.

## Urinary system

- Throughout pregnancy there is an increase in blood supply to the urinary tract in order to cope with the additional demands of the fetus for waste disposal.
- The size and weight of the kidneys increase, whilst the ureters become dilated and elongated to circumvent the enlarging uterus.
- This may cause ureteral reflux or kinking with possible pooling and stagnation of urine leading to an increased risk of urinary tract infections.
- Later on in pregnancy the bladder becomes an intra-abdominal organ, the supporting fascia is stretched and the urethrovesical angle may be altered.
- Pregnant women may therefore complain of frequency, urgency and stress incontinence.

## Musculoskeletal adaptations

- Posture will generally change in pregnancy due to a woman's adaption to the change in the position of her centre of gravity.
- The breasts increase in size by an average of 400–800 g, causing altered thoracic and cervical posture.
- There is a general thought that all spinal curves increase in pregnancy; however Ostgaard et al (1993) found that women generally had an exaggeration of their pre pregnancy posture and those at most risk were those with a naturally large lordosis.
- The distance between the vertical bands of rectus abdominus muscles will widen during pregnancy as the linea alba stretches and sometimes splits.
- A doming of the abdominal muscles occurs during the actions of sitting forward or pulling to get out of bed. Women may need reassurance that this is a normal part of pregnancy. They should be educated about the correct way to get in and out of bed, e.g. rolling onto the side and swinging the legs over the edge of the bed, whilst simultaneously pushing the trunk up using a hand on the bed. This may help to reduce the occurrence of diastasis.
- There is a general increase in water retention resulting in oedema, generally to the dependent areas of the body. This can lead to symptoms of carpal tunnel syndrome as the median and ulnar nerves are compressed. Problems such as facial nerve palsy and meralgia paraesthesia are also seen as a result of pregnancy.
- The common musculoskeletal conditions encountered in WH include:
- Pelvic girdle pain
- Back pain
- Coccydynia
- Carpal tunnel syndrome
- Rectus abdominus divarication.

## Some of the minor ailments associate with pregnancy

- Nausea and vomiting (hyperemesis gravidum).
- Gastro-oesophageal reflux (heartburn).
- Constipation.
- Back and pelvic-girdle pain.
- Carpal tunnel syndrome.

- Haemorrhoids.
- Varicose veins.
- Urinary tract infection.
- Urinary dysfunction – stress and urge incontinence.
- Itching and rashes.
- Painful, enlarged breast.
- Mild breathlessness.
- Headaches.
- Tiredness.
- Insomnia.
- Labile mood.
- Calf cramps.
- Braxton Hicks contractions.

## Assessment

- It is important to understand the normal anatomical, physical and emotional changes that occur in pregnancy and the puerperium in order to understand the abnormal dysfunction that can occur which may lead to pain.
- The physiotherapist will need to draw upon core assessment skills irrespective of the specialist area they work in, with assessment involving history taking, screening and the use of specific tests or measures, and evaluation of the results of examination through analysis and synthesis within a process of clinical reasoning (WCPT 1999).
- A holistic approach to the assessment is important in order to understand the demands both physically and emotionally the woman has in her life.

### Outpatient assessment

#### Subjective assessment

- History of the present complaint (HPC):
- When did it start?
- How?
- 24-hour pattern
- Aggravating and easing movements or activities
- Red flags. Women are equally prone to cauda equina compression and the development of serious pathology as any other woman of equivalent age.
- Obstetric special questions:
- Pain on urination, burning and increased frequency of micturition, potentially due to a urinary tract infection?
- Sudden increase in swelling, particularly face, frontal headache, dizziness, visual disturbance (flashing lights), epigastric pain, nausea and vomiting, due to pre-eclampsia?
- Current obstetric history:
- General health during the pregnancy
- How is care being delivered? Once a woman discovers she is pregnant she will be cared for by either her GP, a community midwifery team, shared care

between her GP and midwifery team or Consultant Obstetrician. Consultant care is usually preserved for those with current or previous complicated pregnancies

– Fetal movements (FM) should be felt after the 20th week of pregnancy in a first pregnancy and around 17/18 weeks in subsequent pregnancies. FM should be felt daily.

- Previous obstetric history:
– Is there a history of musculoskeletal dysfunction in previous pregnancies?
– Type of labour and recovery in the puerperium
– History of postnatal depression?
– These questions may highlight a woman's anxiety about her current pregnancy and may change her perception of any pain.

- Past medical and surgical history:
– Diabetes
– Hypertension
– Previous gynaecological surgery, treatment or endometriosis may have pelvic adhesions causing discomfort as the fetus grows, stretching and compressing pelvic structures. This may cause lower abdominal pain, similar to the stretching of the round ligament
– Previous general surgery
– Pregnant women are not exempt from other health complaints. The older the women is at conception the more likely it is for them to have pre-existing conditions.

- Drug history:
– Many medications are contraindicated in pregnancy
– Women should consult their GP or obstetric consultant regarding which medications are safe for them to take
– There are analgesic medications which are safe to take if guidance is given by a medical practitioner.

- Social history:
– Work/life balance assessment
– Working conditions
– Support at home with ADLs
– Hobbies and sporting activities
– Dependent children.

## Objective assessment

- Assessment starts from the point at which the physiotherapist first observes the woman. Observation of them sitting, standing up and walking into the examination cubicle will start to give an impression of the severity and causative factors of the dysfunction.
- Routine observations include:
– Posture in standing, a raised plinth may be needed for support
– Forward leaning and returning into standing – looking for movement patterns and quality of movement
– Active straight leg raise with and without compression
– Range of movement of joints, noting stiffness and/or pain
– One leg stance – noting movement pattern and pain.

- Women may be able to lie prone with pillows, but may find it more comfortable to side lie or sit in a high forward-leaning position. The physiotherapist should be able to adapt their assessment according to the comfort of the woman.
- The physiotherapist should draw on the core assessment skills when assessing specific joints or areas of the body and seek assistance from a WH or musculoskeletal physiotherapist where appropriate.
- Full neurological assessment should be conducted where clinically appropriate.

## Ward-based assessment

- The role of the WH physiotherapist on the postnatal wards is to encourage recovery after delivery and pregnancy, through education and exercise.
- There are a wide variety of service arrangements across the UK and not all maternity wards will have physiotherapy input.
- WH physiotherapists have to be innovative in the way in which this group of women with very specific needs is cared for.
- Some units will see the majority of woman; some will see those classified as high risk of developing future problems and some women will have no physiotherapeutic intervention.
- Women spend increasingly less time on postnatal wards and therefore it could be argued that physiotherapists would be best placed seeing groups of women in the community at baby clinics, health visitor meetings or other such groups.
- The most important aspect of physiotherapy intervention is that the information and care is delivered with the needs of the woman being central to ensure an effective outcome.

## Early postnatal care

- There are specific issues encountered during the early postnatal period, including:
- Perineal discomfort
- Back or pelvic girdle pain
- Identify those at high risk of developing urinary or faecal incontinence
- High risk of developing urinary or faecal incontinence, due to a forceps delivery, the baby's weight being greater than 4 kg, a prolonged second stage of delivery and a third- or fourth-degree tear.

## Gynaecology

- As part of an obstetric experience students and newly qualified physiotherapists may be required to treat patients after gynaecological surgery.
- This surgery can be minor, e.g. day surgery or involve an overnight stay through to major surgery for gynaecological cancer.
- Some centres will have dedicated gynaecology physiotherapists who will treat the patient holistically, whereas others will have general physiotherapy input either from respiratory or rehabilitation physiotherapists.
- Sometimes women may have attended for out-patient WH physiotherapy treatment, or advice before surgery for stress urinary incontinence or uterine prolapse.

- The material in this volume considers that the approaches described are for specific gynaecological physiotherapy.

## Types of surgery

- To enable effective management of patients' knowledge of the most common investigations and surgical interventions is essential (Table 11.1).

**Table 11.1** Investigations and surgical interventions encountered in gynaecology

| | |
|---|---|
| Bilateral salpingoophorectomy (BSO) | Removal of both ovaries and fallopian tubes |
| Colposcopy | Abnormalities detected on cervical smear<br>A colposcope is a microscope which magnifies the cervix. Biopsies may be taken |
| Cystoscopy | An examination of bladder lining under anaesthetic using a thin 'telescope' inserted into a fluid-filled bladder |
| Debulking | For ovarian tumours, may include removal of ovaries, uterus, cervix and omentum |
| Dilatation and curettage (D&C) | Cervix is dilated and contents or sample of the inner lining of the uterus is removed by suction |
| Hysteroscopy | A thin flexible tube used to look inside the uterus and take a biopsy |
| Inguinal node dissection | Lymph nodes near the vulva are removed following a vulvectomy (unilateral or bilateral) |
| Laparascopy | A telescope enabling the surgeon to view the organs inside the pelvis |
| Laparotomy | Abdominal incision enabling abdominal inspection. Transverse suprapubic incision may be employed (Pfannenstiel). A vertical incision is preferred in ovarian malignancy or for access to the upper abdomen |
| LLETZ | Outpatient treatment for cervical dysplasia (premalignant lesions) aims to remove abnormal cells from the cervix |
| Omenectomy | Removal of the fatty tissue overlying the bowel |
| Pelvic exenteration | For recurrent cancer of the cervix after radiation therapy, tailored to remove the tumour and those organs involved (Hatch and Berek 2005) |
| Pelvic node dissection (PND) | In cases of suspected malignancy, pelvic and para-aortic nodes may be excised |

Continued

| Table 11.1 Continued | |
|---|---|
| Radiotherapy (external/ brachytherapy) | Radiotherapy for gynaecological cancer may be used pre- or postoperatively, as an alternative to surgery, or as palliative treatment |
| Radical total abdominal hysterectomy (RTAH) | Removal of the uterus, fallopian tubes, ovaries, and upper one-third of the vagina |
| Radical trachelectomy | For fertility preservation in patients with early-stage cervical cancer, involves removal of the uterine cervix plus adjacent parametria, conserving the uterine body and ovaries (Grant 2006) |
| Sentinel lymph node biopsy (SLNB) | To locate and assess spread of cancer in the primary lymph node(s) draining lymph from the area in which the cancer developed |
| Subtotal abdominal hysterectomy | Uterus is removed through an incision in the abdominal wall; cervix and ovaries are conserved |
| Total abdominal hysterectomy (TAH) | Removal of the uterus, body and cervix, through an incision in the abdominal wall |
| Vulvectomy | Several stages of vulvectomy exist, including laser surgery for preinvasive abnormal cells, simple vulvectomy when the entire vulva is removed and radical vulvectomy (partial or complete) |

## Preoperative assessment

- Surgery is often complex and a preoperative assessment is recommended (Cook et al 2004).
- This should include:
- Assessment of risk factors, such as obesity, cigarette smoking, debilitative state, previous or planned radiotherapy/chemotherapy, diabetes, chest, heart or circulatory conditions.
- Patient education regarding knowledge and skills for the post-operative and recovery periods.
- Some centres have their own specific literature or use resources provided by Macmillan cancer support (http://www.macmillan.org.uk/Home.aspx).
- Time spent talking to the patient can also be a way of educating them.
- Postoperative assessment, i.e. after the patient has returned to the ward will be the same as for any major surgery.
- The course of the postoperative period depends on the extent of the surgery, pre-existing perimorbid conditions and the development of complications.

## Assessment of outpatients with continence dysfunction

- Risk factors for urinary incontinence include the following:
- Age and gender
- Ethnicity

- Pregnancy and childbirth
- Connective tissue factors
- Smoking, obesity and constipation
- Hysterectomy and urinary incontinence
- Genital prolapse and urinary incontinence
- Radiotherapy and urinary incontinence

---

**Box 11.1** Types of urinary incontinence (ICS/IUGA definitions)

- Urinary incontinence: complaint of involuntary loss of urine
- Stress urinary incontinence: complaint of involuntary loss of urine on effort or physical exertion, or on sneezing or coughing
- Urge urinary incontinence: complaint of involuntary loss of urine associated with urgency
- Postural urinary incontinence: complaint of involuntary loss or urine associated with change of body position, e.g. rising from a seated or lying position
- Nocturnal enuresis: complaint of involuntary urinary loss of urine that occurs during sleep
- Mixed urinary incontinence: complaint of involuntary loss of urine associated with urgency and also with effort or physical exertion or on sneezing or coughing
- Continuous urinary incontinence: complaint of continuous involuntary loss of urine
- Insensible urinary incontinence: complaint of urinary incontinence where the woman has been unaware of how it occurred
- Coital incontinence: complaint of involuntary loss of urine with coitus. This may be further divided into that occurring with penetration and that occurring at orgasm
- Urgency: complaint of a sudden, compelling desire to pass urine which is difficult to defer
- Continence: voluntary control of bladder and bowel function

---

- There are many types of urinary incontinence as defined by the international Continence Society and the International Urogynaecological Association (ICS and IUGA 2009) (Box 11.1).
- As with any condition it is important to establish the exact nature of the problem, i.e. is the problem with storage or emptying, when and how often does it occur, when did it start.
- A full obstetric, medical and surgical history should be documented, along with current drug therapy.
- An essential part of an assessment is a bladder diary enabling the patient to record the time, quantity and type of fluid drunk, the frequency of going to the toilet, the quantity voided and the number of incontinence episodes.
- A 3-day diary is usually recommended to confirm the pattern of day-to-day bladder function.
- Adult fluid output from the kidneys varies between 1 and 3 litres per 24 hours, with approximately 80% excreted during waking hours, negating the need to empty the bladder at night.

- The average adult bladder capacity is in the range 300–600 ml.
- Normal frequency is 6–8 voids in 24 hours.
- Most departments will have a standard pro forma for patients to use.
- To quantify the amount or severity of leakage a pad test is sometimes undertaken, using a preweighed pad.
- The patient usually undertakes a set of exercises which precipitate leakage and then the pad is re-weighed.
- If poor bladder emptying is suspected the measurement of a post-void residual using an ultrasound scanner or in/out catheter should be carried out. Residuals should normally be less than 100 ml.
- Urinalysis should also be undertaken to test for signs of infection, diabetes or haematuria. If any of these tests are abnormal then the patient should be referred to an appropriate specialist.
- A neurological examination should be carried out to test the appropriate dermatomes and myotomes.
- An abdominal examination is undertaken to assess skin condition, surgical incisions including palpation to identify sites of pain, any abnormal pelvic masses, hernias or a distended bladder.
- A physical examination of the external genitalia and pelvic floor muscles (PFM) is essential.
- These assessments require specific training and should only be undertaken following adequate teaching and then under supervision.
- During a vaginal examination, with the patient in crook lying, observations include skin condition, vaginal oestrogenisation status, presence of scars or prolapse (Table 11.2).

**Table 11.2** Examination using the three rings of continence method

| 2 planes of pelvic floor muscle examination (PV) | |
| --- | --- |
| **Vertical plane** | **Horizontal plane** |
| 12 o'clock – symphysis pubis | Finger fully extended |
| 6 o'clock – perineal body | 12 o'clock – coccyx |
| 4 & 8 o'clock – pubococcygeus palpated by distal pad of flexed finger | 6 o'clock – perineal body |
| | 4 & 8 o'clock – pubococcygeus palpated at base of finger |
| | 10 & 2 o'clock – iliococcygeus – distal pad |

- Many of the findings can be recorded on three rings of continence (ROC) representing findings on a vertical and horizontal plane (Figure 11.1).
- The largest ROC represents the vagina, with 12 o'clock denoting the anterior and 6 o'clock the posterior segment; 9 o'clock represents the patient's right lateral wall and 3 o'clock the left.
- The smaller anterior ROC represents the urethra, and the smaller posterior ROC represents the anal canal (Haslam and Laycock 2008).
- During a pelvic floor examination the contraction of the PFM is assessed and often recorded under the acronym PERFECT (Table 11.3) (Laycock and Jerwood 2001).
- This acronym was developed and validated to assess PFM contraction and enable the planning of patient specific muscle training regimens.

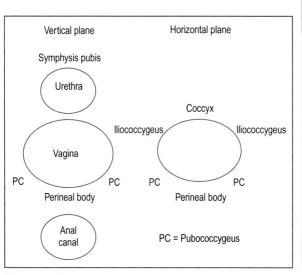

**Figure 11.1** ROC, vertical and horizontal planes.

| Table 11.3 The PERFECT scheme | |
|---|---|
| P Power | A measure of strength of a maximum voluntary contraction |
| E Endurance | The time in seconds the MVC can be held before strength reduces by 50% or more |
| R Repetitions | Number of times the MVC can be repeated |
| F Fast contractions | |
| E Elevation | Lifting of the posterior vaginal wall during a MVC |
| C Co-contraction | Co-contraction of the lower abdominal muscles during an MVC |
| T Timing | Synchronous involuntary contraction of the PFM on coughing |

Example:  P  E  R  F  E  C  T
          3  5  4  7  Y  Y  N

- This assessment describes a patient with a 'normal' (grade 3) Maximal Voluntary Contraction (MVC), held for 5 seconds and repeated 4 times, followed after a rest by 7 fast contractions. In addition elevation of the posterior vaginal wall and co-contraction of the lower abdominals was detected, but involuntary contraction of the PFM on coughing was not demonstrated.
- Aim of treatment here was to increase strength and endurance (repetitions), also more importantly the 'knack'.
- Strength is measured using the Modified Oxford Scale (Table 11.4).

| Table 11.4 Modified Oxford Scale | |
|---|---|
| Grade 0 | No discernible PFM contraction |
| Grade 1 | A flicker, or pulsing under the examining finger, a very weak contraction |
| Grade 2 | A weak contraction – an increase in tension in the muscle without any discernible lift or squeeze |
| Grade 3 | A moderate contraction, characterised by a degree of lifting of the posterior vaginal wall and squeezing on the base of the finger (pubovisceralis) with an indrawing of the perineum. A Grade 3 or higher contraction are generally discernible on visual perineal inspection |
| Grade 4 | A good PFM contraction producing elevation of the posterior vaginal wall against resistance and in-drawing of the perineum. If two fingers are placed laterally in the vagina and separated, a grade 4 contraction can squeeze them together against resistance |
| Grade 5 | A strong contraction of the PFM; strong resistance can be given against elevation of the posterior vaginal wall and approximation of the index and middle fingers as above |

- Assessment of the PFM may also be undertaken using electromyography, which is the extracellular recording of bio-electrical activity generated by muscle fibres.
- Surface EMG, using intravaginal or anal devices may be used.
- Vaginal squeeze pressure measurement and transperineal or transabdominal ultrasound imaging are two further methods of assessing and providing feedback to patients.

## Bowel dysfunction

- Requires a detailed medical, surgical and obstetric history.
- It is important to find out about the history of symptoms:
- Usual bowel pattern and consistency
- Urgency with an ability to defer defecation
- Presence of urge or passive incontinence/soiling
- Presence of blood and mucus
- Ability to control flatulence, or pain.
- It is also important to establish the presence of defecation difficulties such as having to sit on the toilet a long time, straining, use of digital stimulation, feeling of obstructed defecation.
- A list of medications taken by the patient should be established and these should include over-the-counter medications as well as those prescribed.
- Other factors which need to be recorded are the patient's diet, if they smoke, their weight, any recent changes, fluid intake, skin problems, and the effect of their bowel dysfunction on their lifestyle and relationships.

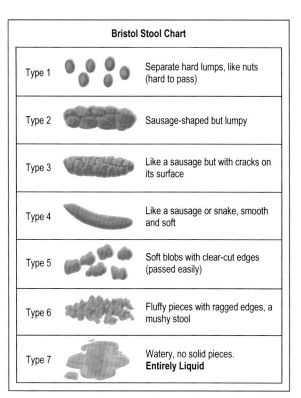

**Figure 11.2** Bristol Stool Chart.

- A bowel diary is also an essential part of the assessment for those patients with bowel symptoms. This will record the frequency of defecation, stool type (Figure 11.2) and soiling episodes (Lewis and Heaton 1997).
- A physical examination should include inspection of the perianal skin, of the perineum for scarring from episiotomy or obstetric tears, inspection of the posterior wall of the vagina for any rectocele, perineal descent, presence of a loaded rectum and a digital examination of the anal canal to determine resting and squeeze tone.
- This should only be performed following appropriate training.
- Constipation is present if patients who do not take laxatives report at least two of the following in any 12-week period during the previous 12 months (Rome Foundation 2010):
- Fewer than three bowel movements per week
- Hard stool in more that 25% of bowel movements
- A sense of incomplete evacuation in more than 25%

- Excessive straining in more than 25%
- A need for digital manipulation to facilitate evacuation.
- Functional constipation can either be slow-transit constipation, where there is delayed transit through the colon and rectum, or obstructed defecation, but not outlet obstruction, associated with advancing age. This includes syndromes such as descending peroneum, dyssynergia (anismus) and anterior rectal wall prolapse.

## Prolapse

- Genital prolapse or pelvic organ prolapse (POP) refers to a loss of fibromuscular support of the pelvic viscera resulting in a vaginal protrusion.
- The prolapse is usually described according to the area of the vagina in which it occurs.
- Anterior vaginal prolapse generally involves the bladder (cystocele) and often involves hypermobility of the urethrovesical junction as well.
- Posterior vaginal prolapse can involve the rectum (rectocele), small bowel (enterocele) or the sigmoid colon (sigmoidocele).
- Apical prolapse describes loss of the support at the apex of the vagina.
- Vaginal vault prolapse refers to a complete or partial inversion of the vaginal apex usually found in patients who have had a hysterectomy.
- Prevalence: 50% of parous women have some degree of prolapse, but only 10 to 20% seek evaluation.
- There is multifactorial aetiology, including pregnancy and childbirth, hormonal factors, constipation, smoking, obesity, exercise, previous pelvic surgery.
- Most women complain of feeling discomfort or heaviness within the pelvis in addition to a 'lump coming down'.
- Symptoms tend to become worse with prolonged standing and towards the end of the day.
- They may also complain of dyspareunia, difficulty in inserting tampons and chronic low back ache.
- In cases of third-degree prolapse there may be epithelial ulceration and lichenification, which results in a symptomatic vaginal discharge or bleeding. These may be associated with lower urinary tract (LUT) symptoms of urgency and frequency in addition to a sensation of incomplete emptying.
- Posterior vaginal wall prolapse may be associated with difficulty in opening the bowels.
- Assessment.
- Similar to continence assessment, or pelvic organ prolapse – quantification (POP-Q) (Hagen and Stark 2008).

## Pelvic pain

- Chronic pelvic pain has been defined as 'non-malignant pain perceived in structures related to the pelvis of either men or women'.
- Pelvic pain syndrome has a separate definition proposed by Abrams et al (2002) and adopted by Fall et al (2004) as the 'occurrence of persistent or recurrent episodic pelvic pain associated with symptoms suggestive of lower urinary tract, sexual, bowel or gynaecological dysfunction'.

- There is no proven infection or other obvious pathology.
- The true prevalence and incidence of PFM pain syndrome alone or coexisting with other chronic pelvic pain conditions is unknown.
- They are complex and challenging conditions with a significant lack of evidence underpinning the basic elements of PFM therapy for pelvic pain or muscle over-activity.
- A comprehensive assessment should incorporate a bio-psychosocial approach.
- The PFM should be evaluated for the presence of over-activity, trigger points, and reduced elasticity.
- The aim of assessment is to reproduce and quantify the patient's symptoms.

## Consent

- Each department should have an agreed policy on the consent required prior to any intimate examination.
- It is essential to obtain and record valid consent (some institutions require written consent) and with any refusal recorded.
- The GMC has published guidance for doctors undertaking intimate examinations (GMC 2006).
- Clinical guidelines for the Physiotherapy Management of Females aged 16–65 years with stress urinary incontinence are available from the CSP (Laycock and Jerwood 2001).

The references for this chapter can be found on www.expertconsult.com.

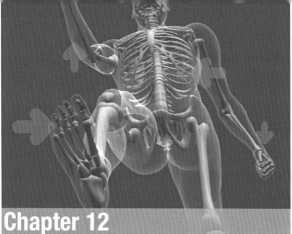

# Chapter 12
# Oncology and Palliative Care

## Introduction

- The primary aim of physiotherapy in oncology and palliative care is to reduce the effects of the disease and to maximize independence with regard to physical, psychosocial and economic function.

- Physiotherapeutic objectives vary, being determined by a holistic approach to assessment (physical, psychological, social and spiritual) and goal setting in partnership with the patient (Wood-Dauphinee and Küchler 1992, ACPOPC 1993).

- A holistic approach in oncology and palliative care is particularly important as patients tend to have a complex mix of symptoms and problems that may not be physical in nature. It is imperative that the physiotherapist considers how each of the patient's problems link together, e.g. how anxiety may influence breathlessness.

- Goal setting is essential, with goals being reviewed relative to a patient's changing condition, to maintain hope, increase confidence and to achieve a feeling of success, especially towards the end stages of life.

- Working in an oncology and palliative care environment can be emotionally demanding. The physiotherapist may often face sensitive situations where advanced communication skills are vital.

- If the physiotherapist is unable to answer questions from a patient they must seek advice from a senior member of staff.

## Preparation for assessment

- In an inpatient setting medical notes will be a source of information about the history of the patient.

- The physiotherapist will need to explore the current history, previous history, social history, drug history and consider any recent test results e.g. blood results, MRI scans, X-rays, myotome testing and dermatomal testing.

- It is important to know normal values for tests and how results may influence a patient's condition (Appendix 12.1).

- Before beginning the assessment discuss the case with the multidisciplinary team (MDT), to gain useful information and insight about the patient.

- In an outpatient or community setting, access the patient's notes, which will contain clinic review reports, test results and plans for treatment.

- Find out how much the patient knows about their diagnosis and how much they want to know.

- Some patients use denial as a coping mechanism and it is important that this is respected.

- In some cases it may be the family who do not want the diagnosis or prognosis disclosed. To avoid colluding with family members the physiotherapist should discuss the situation with the MDT and get a consensus on how this should be managed.

- A physiotherapist should always discuss any concerns that they may have about communicating with the patient or relatives with a senior colleague.

- The physiotherapist should know why the patient has been referred, but allow the patient to express their concerns and problems.

- Discharge planning should start from the day the patient is admitted and should involve the MDT, including the hospital discharge co-ordinator.

- The physiotherapist needs to attend regular team meetings and case conferences, recognizing the needs and expectations of the patient.

## Subjective assessment

### Observations and values

- In the in-patient setting it may be important to check observations such as heart rate, blood pressure and blood values.

- With many oncology and palliative care patients, these normal values may be at the lower or higher ends and this does not necessarily preclude physiotherapy intervention.

- The physiotherapist should be aware of any relevant local policies or guidelines.

### Communication

- Ensure adequate time and privacy have been allocated.

- The physiotherapist should introduce themselves to the patient and explain their role, sitting down if possible to indicate that they have time to listen.

- Open questions should be used to encourage the patient to talk, e.g. 'How are you today?' rather than 'how is your pain?'

- It is essential to establish what the patient knows about their condition, a useful phrase might be 'Can you tell me about what has been happening to you?'

- In an outpatient/community setting where the patient has been referred for a specific problem, it is important to give the patient the opportunity to share other problems too, e.g. 'You have been referred by your consultant for… (the specific problem). How are you today?' or 'Have you any other difficulties that I may be able to help with?' these openings provide the patient with the opportunity to raise other concerns.

- Ask the patient to prioritize their problems, if they have several, e.g. 'What are your three biggest problems at the moment, starting with the one that is the most troublesome for you?' This gives the patient the opportunity to highlight concerns from their point of view rather than the impersonal way that they can be listed in the medical notes.

- The patient should be encouraged to express their feelings, e.g. it may be appropriate to ask 'what worries you most about your situation?' Attending to verbal cues can help the physiotherapist to identify and explore a patient's anxieties.

- For example:

  'I don't want to die the way my father did.'

  'Can you tell me what you mean by that?'

  'Well, he died struggling for breath and it was very frightening.'

- Reflecting the question back to the patient may allow deeper exploration of concerns, which can then be discussed.

- For example

  'Do you think I'll ever walk again?'

  'What makes you ask that question?'

  'Well, I'm wondering what my future will be like if I can't walk.'

- It may be useful to summarize what the patient has just said from time to time and feed back to the patient, to check for accuracy and allow clarification of any misunderstanding.

- For example:

  'Can I just check, when you said you would like to go home, did you mean for the weekend or are you talking about the long term?'

- One of the most challenging tasks for a physiotherapist in oncology and palliative care is achieving the right balance between professional honesty and maintaining hope during communication.

- It is best to give a more generalized answer to questions initially and then check for the patient's response, with a more detailed answer being given if the patient requests more information.

- If the patient stops in the middle of a sentence, repeating the last three words back to them may encourage them to continue.

- For example

  'Sometimes I feel …' (pause)

  'Sometimes you feel …'

  'Sometimes I feel that I might not walk again.'

- The physiotherapist should avoid filling silences with conversation. Silence may feel uncomfortable or lengthy to the physiotherapist, but it is likely that the patient will find such pauses a useful opportunity to think.

- The physiotherapist may not always know the answer to a question and it is important to acknowledge this, explaining to the patient that you will ask the most appropriate person to answer the question to come and speak with them.

- A patient's information needs vary considerably during the course of their illness and it is important to be mindful of this.
- Some patients manage to live parallel realities, having the capacity to acknowledge the serious nature of their illness, yet hope for a cure or remission. Others can appear to have full insight and acceptance one day and be in denial the next, oscillating back and forth throughout the course of their illness. Accept a patient's insight as it presents on a day-to-day basis.
- Having exchanged the necessary information, the patient and the physiotherapist can agree goals.
- Goals need to be relevant to the individual patient and in some cases they may need to be short term. If a goal seems unattainable, break it down into smaller goals. This is more likely to foster a feeling of success for the patient.
- Let the patient know that the conversation is coming to a close, this provides them with an opportunity to ask any other questions. 'We have covered a lot of ground, is there anything else you would like to ask?'

## Red and yellow flags

- 'Red flags' may be identified that warrant further medical assessment.
- 'Yellow flags' often indicate psychosocial risks, which entail further assessment and specific treatment interventions (Appendix 12.2).

## Goal setting

- Following subjective assessment, goals need to be set with the patient.
- Goals need to be specific and personal to the individual (Bovend'Eerdt et al 2009).
- SMART goals can be set (Table 12.1), with involvement of the family or carers if the patient consents to this.
- To ensure effective multidisciplinary team-working the MDT need to be aware of the goals.

## Outcome measures

- Clinical outcome measures should be valid, reliable, sensitive and relevant to a patient's individual clinical needs and treatment goals, taking into account their status and care setting. (Appendix 12.3).

## Assessment of specific symptoms or problems

### Breathlessness

- Twycross (2003) defined 'breathlessness as the subjective experience of breathing discomfort'.
- Breathlessness is 'subjective, like pain, it involves both perception of the sensation by the patient and his reaction to the sensation' (Heyse-Moore et al 1991).
- The patient's emotional state and other symptoms can have a direct impact on the symptom of breathlessness.

**Table 12.1** SMART goal setting

| | |
|---|---|
| **S**pecific | The goal should be specific to the individuals needs |
| | The goal is discussed with the patient to understand why it is important to them |
| | The patient's diagnosis, prognosis, social background and timing of treatment intervention must be considered when setting the goals |
| **M**easurable | The physiotherapist and the patient must be able to measure success |
| | It is essential the physiotherapist uses a repeatable outcome measure to show the efficacy of treatment, to guide clinical decisions and further goal setting |
| **A**ttainable | Goals should challenge the patient, but at the same time need to be achievable. Starting with short-term goals will allow the patient to maintain their motivation and then longer-term goals can be set |
| **R**ealistic | This is often the most challenging part when setting goals. The physiotherapist may need to negotiate with the patient and family/carers to ensure goals are not unrealistic. If goals are not going to be achieved it will cause frustration and upset for the patient especially |
| **T**imely | The goal should have a clear start date and the physiotherapist should use reflections with the patient to show progression |
| | The goals should be set at the most appropriate time of the patient's condition and reviewed on a regular basis |
| | A written diary may be useful to allow the patient to see written evidence of their progression |

## Assessment

- A respiratory assessment is undertaken, considering the diagnosis, treatment and care setting.
- The specifics of the assessment will vary, e.g. in an acute ward setting, a patient diagnosed with cancer may present with a chest infection, therefore it would be appropriate to auscultate the chest, check oxygen saturation levels and to observe the pattern and work of breathing. In a palliative care setting where a patient has advanced lung cancer, it is appropriate to focus on the breathing pattern and technique, considering factors influencing the breathlessness such as anxiety.
- Each patient must be assessed on an individual basis.
- The most commonly used outcome measures for breathlessness are the Modified Borg Scale (Box 12.1) and the Visual Analogue Scale (Figure 13.1, Chapter 13). Both are reasonably simple to use and most patients can understand them (Wilson and Jones 1989).

## Exercise tolerance/deconditioning

- Weakness, fatigue and deconditioning due to lack of exercise are common problems.

| **Box 12.1** Modified Borg Scale | |
|---|---|
| 0 | Nothing at all |
| 0.5 | Very, very slight, just noticeable |
| 1 | Very slight |
| 2 | Slight |
| 3 | Moderate |
| 4 | Somewhat severe |
| 5 | Severe |
| 6 | Severe |
| 7 | Very severe |
| 8 | Very severe |
| 9 | Very, very severe, almost maximal |
| 10 | Maximal |

- Cancer treatments are toxic to the body and can result in marked loss of physical function.
- Patients in palliative care settings can have significant muscle weakness and mobility issues. The complexity of combined symptoms can be challenging, e.g. cachexia which affects muscle mass and exercise tolerance as a result of derangement in the body's metabolism, due to a tumour or by the response of the body to a tumour such as cytokine activity (Hawkins 2007).
- Activity has been proven to be beneficial for cancer patients and the assumption that rest will help increase energy levels and exercise tolerance should be challenged (Hawkins 2007).

### Assessment of de-conditioning and exercise tolerance

- Cancer patients may receive physiotherapy at any stage of their illness and in various clinical settings.
- Assessment for the level of de-conditioning will include multiple factors (Box 12.2).
- It is generally accepted that platelet levels should be above $20 \times 10^9$/L for gentle exercise and $50 \times 10^9$/L for increase in physical activity using resistance.
- Neutrophil levels should be greater than $0.5 \times 10^9$/L in order to avoid exposure to infection (Rankin et al 2008) (Appendix 12.1).
- Patients undergoing treatment are especially subject to physical and psychological change as they respond to therapeutic regimens (Schneider et al 2003).
- Assessment should include awareness of complications and avoid exacerbating the cytotoxic effects of treatments (Appendix 12.4).
- In palliative care, the assessment should be adjusted according to disease and increasing fragility, caused by exacerbating symptoms such as bony metastases and ascites.
- With a deteriorating condition the aim of treatment will be to maintain function, stamina, mobility and quality of life, in addition to controlling symptoms.

> **Box 12.2** Considerations when assessing deconditioning and exercise tolerance
>
> - Cancer history, including site and stage of cancer
> - Current treatment, drugs and side effects, time of administration
> - Past medical history
> - Previous activity levels and current exercise tolerance, timed walk test
> - Cardiovascular assessment, resting heart rate, CV potential
> - Pulmonary function and oxygen saturation
> - Muscle power 0–5 (Medical Research Council scale)
> - Range of movement and flexibility
> - Assessment of neurological problems
> - Balance
> - Fatigue
> - Nutritional status and gastrointestinal status
> - Psychosocial status

## Fatigue

- Cancer-related fatigue (CRF) is a complex multifactorial symptom affecting many patients in all phases of the disease.
- It has been described as a common persistent and subjective sense of tiredness related to cancer or to cancer treatment that interferes with usual functioning.
- 70–100% of cancer patients experience CRF (Lundh et al 2006).

### Assessment of CRF

- The subjective sense of tiredness can be difficult to assess to get an accurate picture of how a patient is being affected.
- It is common in oncology and palliative care.
- The NCAT Rehabilitation Pathways (2009a, b) for Fatigue and Energy Management provide a framework for evaluating the effects of CRF. It is based on a Visual Analogue Scale of 0–10, 10 being the worst fatigue, with a score of 4 and above requiring specialist multidisciplinary intervention. Scores below 4 should be informed about coping strategies.
- The International Classification of Diseases has developed criteria to aid CRF diagnosis (Box 12.3).
- Fatigue is also a common symptom of depression and if suspected should be referred for appropriate assessment.
- Fatigue measurement tools are essential to assess both the fatigue itself and outcomes of interventions.
- Effort is required to complete the assessment tasks. In the palliative setting a shorter scale may be more appropriate.
- There are a range of commonly used outcome measures for measuring fatigue (Appendix 12.3).

**Box 12.3** Criteria of cancer-related fatigue

- Symptoms:
- Significant fatigue
- Diminished energy
- Increased need to rest, disproportionate to any recent change in activity level
- Plus 6 or more of the following:
- General weakness or heaviness of limbs
- Diminished concentration
- Decreased motivation or interest in usual activities
- Insomnia or hypersomnia
- Experience of sleep as un-refreshing or non-restorative
- Perceived need to struggle to overcome inactivity
- Marked emotional reactivity to feeling fatigued, e.g. sadness, frustration, irritability
- Difficulty completing tasks due to feeling fatigued
- Perceived problems with short-term memory
- Post exertional malaise lasting several hours
- These symptoms are not considered to be a consequence of other conditions (Cella et al 2001)

## Lymphoedema

- An accumulation of fluid and other elements (e.g. protein) in tissue spaces, as a result of imbalance between interstitial fluid production and transport (usually a low-output failure). It may manifest as swelling of one or more limbs including the corresponding quadrant of the trunk. Swelling may also be found in other areas, e.g. head and neck, breast and genitalia (Lymphoedema Framework 2006).
- Caused by congenital dysplasia, (primary lymphoedema) or anatomical obliteration, e.g. after radical operations, such as axilla or retroperitoneal nodal sampling, irradiation or repeated lymphangitis (ISL 2009).
- Lymphoedema is incurable and prompt treatment is required to manage signs and symptoms effectively. The patients at risk need to be identified if they develop signs and symptoms and referred to local and regional services via the MDT (Box 12.4).

**Box 12.4** Signs and symptoms of lymphoedema

- Feeling of heaviness, tightness, fullness or stiffness
- Clothing or jewellery may become tight
- Aching
- Observable swelling
- Skin marking from underwear

### Assessment of lymphoedema

- Lymphoedema may present at any time following a diagnosis or treatment for cancer.

| Table 12.2 | Lymphoedema staging (adapted from ISL 2009) |
|---|---|
| Stage 0 | A subclinical state |
| Stage 1 | Fluid in tissues resolves on elevation and pitting may be seen |
| Stage 2 | Manifest pitting, no reduction in elevation |
| Late Stage 2 | Oedema firm, pitting may not be evident |
| Stage 3 | Hard, thickened skin, no pitting, skin folds, fat deposits, warty growths, hyperpigmentation |

- The physiotherapist should be able to identify signs of lymphoedema, these might include:
- History and/or physical and functional assessment
- History of infection and cellulitis
- Assessment of swelling, including shape of limb and if an adjacent quadrant affected
- Scarring and subcutaneous changes such as fibrosis and tissue thickening
- Posture and positioning
- Pain
- Basic skin condition, e.g. dryness, colour, temperature, fragility, fungal infection, hyperkeratosis
- Lymphorrhoea – lymph leakage through the skin
- Signs of acute infection, e.g. hot, painful red swelling with or without flu-like symptoms.
- The patient should be made aware of risk factors, signs and symptoms of cellulitis or lymphoedema and the appropriate action to take (see Box 12.4).
- The physiotherapist may be required to measure limb volumes and should follow local procedures and seek advice of an experienced colleague prior to carrying this out.
- Consideration must be given to other causes of oedema such as DVT, CCF, dependency, chronic venous insufficiency, recurrence of cancer, and other organ dysfunctions.
- A diagnosis of lymphoedema should necessitate a referral to local/regional lymphoedema services where a further more detailed assessment would occur.
- This would include staging (Table 12.2), specialist investigations, limb volumes, skin condition, presence of Stemmer's sign, skin folds, BMI, pain and psychosocial assessment.

## Mobility

- Evidence suggests that there is a positive association between physical activity and quality of life (Lowe et al 2009, Helbostad et al 2009).
- A decline in physical function has been linked with the patient's awareness of their own terminality causing psychological distress and affecting decision-making in end-of-life care (Gauthier and Swigart 2003).
- Most oncology and palliative care patients experience; fatigue, pain, dyspnoea and nausea, and may have concurrent co-morbidities which contribute to reduce physical activity and function.

- Patients need appropriate rehabilitation in order to function at a minimum level of dependency and optimize their quality of life, regardless of life expectancy.
- Mobility becomes more challenging as disease progresses and the physiotherapist can help the patient and carers decide which activities they can realistically perform, within the limits of energy, safely and capabilities.

## Assessment of mobility

- Check for attachments, such as drips, peripherally inserted central catheters (PICC line), syringe drivers or urinary catheters.
- The subjective assessment may give insight into the patient's mobility history.
- It may be useful to enquire about:
- The patient's premorbid mobility status
- The patient's recent/current mobility status
- Whether the patient perceives mobility to be improving or deteriorating?
- If there is a history of falls
- If the patient experiences changes in blood pressure or postural hypotension
- What the patient identifies as the most troublesome aspects of mobility
- Whether the patient has been prescribed any mobility aids/wheelchair.
- The key elements of the assessment are similar to a mobility assessment in any other setting and will include: bed mobility, sit to stand, transfers, balance, gait, the ability to manage stairs and overall function.
- It is essential to be aware of symptoms that may restrict mobility, e.g. pain, fatigue, bone metastases, nausea and vomiting, dyspnoea, lymphoedema, steroid-induced muscle weakness, postural hypotension, continence problems or cognitive ability.
- Due to the diverse range of conditions that are common in oncology and palliative care patients, it may be appropriate to conduct a neurological, musculoskeletal or respiratory assessment in conjunction with a mobility assessment. There are a wide variety of outcome measures that are suitable for oncology and palliative care patients (Appendix 12.3).

## Conditions and associated neurological signs and symptoms

### Metastatic spinal cord compression (MSCC)

- MSCC is an oncological emergency, requiring precise assessment of symptoms, urgent investigations and immediate treatment.
- The physiotherapist must have an understanding of spinal cord compression to complete a thorough assessment.
- Evidence suggests that 10% of patients who had no prior malignant diagnosis, will present with MSCC as their first manifestation of cancer and that in 70% of cases compression occurs in the thoracic spine, 20% in the lumbar spine and 10% in the cervical spine (Perrin et al 1997).
- Pain in usually the earliest symptom of a MSCC, often presenting as a band-like pain which corresponds with the level of compression, other signs are:
- Radicular pain
- Limb weakness
- Difficulty walking

- Sensory loss
- Bladder or bowel dysfunction.
- Any patient suspected with a spinal cord compression must remain on full spinal precautions until medical assessment and correct clinical imaging have been carried out.
- The preferred imaging is an MRI scan unless there are specific contraindications.

## Assessment

- A neurological baseline assessment is required (Appendix 12.5).
- Recovery following a cord compression is dependent upon the individual, e.g. patients who present with significantly decreased neurology at the point of diagnosis may have less chance of recovering full motor function.
- It is only when spinal stability has been assessed and confirmed that the patient can start to sit up in bed with close monitoring for changes in neurology/symptoms (Table 12.3).
- If a patient shows any signs of deteriorating neurology they should be laid flat and a spinal surgery opinion sought.
- The physiotherapist must always work within their level of competency and seek further advice from senior staff as necessary (NICE 2008).
- Key aims of rehabilitation with MSCC patients during pre treatment stage:
- Immobilization of spine
- Baseline assessment of neurological function
- Prevention of respiratory and/or circulatory problems
- Pain relief
- Maintenance of joint ROM
- Education, information and support.

| Table 12.3 Spinal cord compression checklist |
| --- |
| Physiotherapist Introduction |
| Establishing patients knowledge and understanding |
| **Assessment** |
| Muscle charting |
| Sensation |
| Pain – neuropathic/mechanical |
| Tone |
| Range of movement |
| Dermatomes |
| Respiratory assessment |
| Aims for rehabilitation |

## Brain and spinal cord tumours

- There are two main types of brain tumour, primary and secondary (metastatic), they account for less than 2% of all cancer diagnoses in the UK.

- Within the group of primary brain tumours there are nearly 100 different types of tumour, generally named after the type of cell they developed from.
- The common descriptions of primary brain tumours are either 'benign' or 'malignant'.
- Benign tumours, although slow-growing and less likely to reoccur if removed, can still transform into more aggressive tumours, or cause significant damage dependant on their location. Malignant tumours, also known as 'high grade' tend to be faster growing and may spread further into the brain or spinal cord.
- Primary brain tumours very rarely spread outside the central nervous system.
- The common types, grading and prognosis of brain tumours are listed in Appendix 12.6.
- Patients can present with a variety of symptoms dependent on the type, location and nature of the tumour.
- Patients also have the potential to change very quickly, particularly the high-grade primary brain tumours.
- Intradural spinal cord tumours are rare and are classified as extramedullary (arising inside the dura but outside the spinal cord) or intramedullary (originating in the spinal cord).
- The most common extramedullary tumours are schwannomas and meningiomas, with ependymomas and astrocytomas arising from the cord itself.
- Primary lymphoma is another extramedullary tumour, but is extremely rare.
- Spinal tumours can often present with a protracted history of pain and associated neurological dysfunction below the level of the tumour.
- Physiotherapists working in a musculoskeletal setting may encounter such patients pre-diagnosis and need to be aware of red flags (Appendix 12.2).
- High-grade tumours in the cord carry a poor prognosis with an average life expectancy of between 6 and 12 months (NICE 2006).
- Low-grade tumours may have a better outlook in terms of longevity, although they will often have resulting disability and functional problems.

## Assessment

- Assessment will depend on the patient's condition and the setting, but should include a neurological assessment, particularly in the acute setting after surgery (if applicable) to obtain baseline measurements.
- In other settings, or at different stages of the pathway, it may be more appropriate to focus on a functional assessment of movement and ability, dependent on the individual patient.
- Patients with a brain or spinal cord tumour should be assessed as any other neurologically presenting patient (such as CVA) but taking into consideration that the patient may fatigue more quickly and the assessment may need to take place over several sessions.
- These patients may also be suffering from increased levels of pain and this must be taken into account in planning the assessment.

## Plexopathy

- Tumour infiltration as a result of disease progression and radiation injury are the most common causes of plexopathy in oncology and palliative care (Reddy 2006).

- Symptoms include pain, loss of motor control, sensory deficits and an overall deterioration in function.
- Brachial plexopathy is most commonly associated with lymphoma, and breast and lung cancers. Pain is the predominant presenting feature, often preceding the onset of focal neurological signs by several months.
- Tumour invasion of the lower cords is more common, e.g. Pancoast syndrome (due to apical lung cancer), than invasion of the upper cords, giving rise to neurological signs and symptoms in the distribution of C8 to T1 roots.
- Radiation injury is more commonly associated with the upper cords.
- Lumbosacral plexopathy is often associated with genitourinary, gynaecological and colonic cancers. Pain varies with the site of plexus involvement. Radicular pain may present in the L1 to L3 distribution (anterior aspect of the thigh and groin) or in the L5–S1 distribution (posterior aspect of the leg to the heel). Sometimes, only referred pain is present, commonly in the anterior aspect of the thigh, the knee and the lateral aspect of the calf.

## Peripheral neuropathy

- Peripheral neuropathy is usually caused by damage to nerves from surgery, radiation treatment, or chemotherapy.
- It can also be caused by a tumour pressing on or penetrating a nerve.
- Chemotherapy-induced peripheral neuropathy as a result of neurotoxicity is a complication most commonly associated with the cytotoxic drugs vinca alkaloids, platinum-based compounds and taxols, and the degree of reversibility is variable. The extent of neurological damage depends on the drug used, the duration of treatment and the cumulative dose applied (Quasthoff and Hartung 2002).
- Symptoms vary widely and may adversely affect quality of life.
- Patients may present with muscle weakness, distal paraesthesia, allodynia and muscle cramps.

## Progressive neurological conditions

- Many patients will have palliative care needs, most commonly those diagnosed with more aggressive conditions, e.g. motor neuron disease (MND), multiple systems atrophy (MSA) or progressive supranuclear palsy (PSP).
- Patients with other conditions such as multiple sclerosis and Parkinson's disease may also access palliative care services towards the end of their disease process or if there are complex symptom management issues.

### Assessment

- It is vital to assess the key functions that the patient may find difficult, such as bed mobility, toileting and hand function for eating and dressing, etc.
- With conditions such as MND, MSA and PSP the patients can deteriorate quickly and therefore reassessment at regular intervals is essential to provide optimum care.
- It is important to include family and carers in the assessment process, particularly if they will be providing care and assistance to the patient or they will be required to assist in physiotherapy programmes.

## Pain

- Pain can be described as 'an unpleasant sensory or emotional experience associated with actual or potential tissue damage' (IASP 1994).
- It is a complex phenomenon being the culmination of several factors, physical or non-physical.
- A multidimensional, multiprofessional approach is needed to address the psychological, social and spiritual effects of pain.
- Physiotherapists have an important role to play in the management of this distressing symptom and should use a holistic, flexible, patient-focused approach, to conduct a comprehensive assessment and to implement treatment (Robb and Ewer-Smith 2008).
- The concept of total pain (Figure 12.1) was developed in the 1960s by Dane Cicely Saunders, emphasizing the multidimensional aspects of pain (Clark 1999).

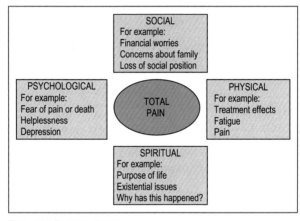

**Figure 12.1** Total pain diagram.

### Assessment

- A pain history will give insight into the background and the development of a patient's pain.
- It is important to differentiate between the assessment and measurement of pain.
- Assessment is 'the broader examination of the relationship between different components of the pain experience, for a given patient', whereas measurement is 'the quantification of each component' (Strong et al 2002).
- The essential components of a physiotherapy assessment include a description of the pain, responses to the pain and the impact of the pain on a patient's life. The latter can be assessed by exploring functional limitation and physical impairments.
- Assessment is unlikely to take place in a single interaction, but information is usually gathered over a series of patient contacts.

- A holistic pain assessment should include medical and psychosocial history (including recognition of spiritual, cultural and religious aspects).

- Throughout the assessment and subsequent treatment, physiotherapists must remain vigilant for 'red flags' which may indicate disease progression (Appendix 12.2).

- It is important to bear in mind that two thirds of cancer patients have more than one pain and a third have three or more pains (Twycross 2003).

- Assessment will assist the identification of priorities and the goals of treatment, interventions recommended and likely outcomes with timescales.

- Any likely adverse effects of treatment should be clearly explained to the patient.

- The use of a pain diary may provide insight into:

- The nature of the pain, e.g. neuropathic

- The characteristics of the pain, e.g. location, duration, radiation, severity, constant/intermittent

- Diurnal variations

- Triggers

- Aggravating activities and impacts on lifestyle

- The impact of psychological and spiritual factors

- Medications taken/other treatments tried/positional adjustments and their effects.

## Range of movement (ROM) problems

- Decreased joint range can be caused by surgery, side effects from treatment, de-conditioning or the disease itself.

- Assessment may be required for a specific problem, e.g. a shoulder or neck following breast surgery.

- In the case of the palliative patient the assessment of ROM may take place through functional movements and/or mobility assessment when pain is controlled.

### Assessment

- There are many factors to consider when carrying out a routine assessment of ROM.

- These include tissue extensibility, muscle shortening, spasms, scarring, radiation fibrosis, cording and any other presenting symptoms (Figure 12.2).

- Some of these symptoms may limit assessment and may need addressing before the physiotherapist can fully evaluate potential.

## Psychological aspects

### Anxiety and depression

- Fear and anxiety are normal reactions to the stress of undergoing cancer treatment.

- Depression is when a patient's mood is low most of the time for several weeks or more. The relationship between cancer and depression is complex and multifactorial.

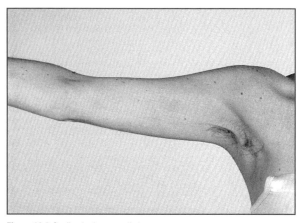

**Figure 12.2** Cording in the upper limb.

## Assessment

- It is important to be aware of the issues of anxiety and depression in order to identify patients who may need referral on to a specialist.
- Common presentations can be; breathlessness, muscle tension, dizziness, sweating and panic attacks.
- Depression can express itself in a patient who has no motivation, expresses helplessness or hopelessness or guilt and blame.
- Anxiety and depression assessment scales are used, e.g. Hospital Anxiety and Depression Scale (HADS) or Brief Edinburgh Depression Scale (BEDS).
- Both provide a method of screening for anxiety and depression (Appendix 12.3).

## Body image

- This is our own impression of our physical appearance and what sort of person we feel we are. This image is built up over time from observing ourselves, the reactions of others, and a complex interaction of attitudes, emotions, memories, fantasies and experiences (Regnard and Kindlen 2002).
- Our body image is also affected by social interactions and how we relate to others, our feelings of achievement and self worth, our sexual image of attractiveness and our spirituality and morality.

- Cancer and its treatment can produce temporary and permanent changes which can have a devastating effect on patients' feelings and their attitude towards their body, which can affect their psychological health.

## Assessment

- Physiotherapists should be aware of body image issues.
- Listening to a patient's concerns is of paramount importance. Often an open discussion and acknowledgement can bring down barriers, reduce feelings of isolation and fear of rejection.
- Referral to formal body image services or psychological support may be required and should be a MDT decision (Appendix 12.3).

## Hope

- 'A multidimensional dynamic life force, characterized by a confident yet uncertain expectation of achieving future good, which, to the hoping person is realistically possible and personally significant' (Dufault and Martocchio 1985).
- Fostering hope and preventing feelings of abandonment are part of the physiotherapeutic intervention (Doyle et al 2005).
- Patients need attainable goals to help maintain a sense of control and to reframe a vision for the future. Some patients choose to avoid receiving information in order to maintain hope.
- Honesty, empathy, optimism and excellent communication skills are required to assist the patient.
- Kylma et al (2009) identified key factors contributing to and threatening hope in palliative care (Table 12.4).

**Table 12.4** Hope, supporting factors and threats

| Factors supporting hope | Factors threatening hope |
| --- | --- |
| Attainable goals that help to maintain a sense of control | Physical or emotional loss |
| Affirmation of worth | Losing the future |
| Honest information | Loss of healthcare professional's interest |
| Symptom management | Devaluation of personhood |
| Trust in care | |

## Specific issues related to tumour sites

- Issues or symptoms related to the common tumour sites types are shown in Table 12.5.

The references for this chapter can be found on www.expertconsult.com.

**Table 12.5** Issues related to specific tumour sites

| Symptoms | Breast | Head & Neck | Lung | Colorectal | Upper GI | Gynaecology | Brain/CNS | Sarcoma | Haematology | Skin | Urology |
|---|---|---|---|---|---|---|---|---|---|---|---|
| Bleeding | | | ✓ | ✓ | ✓ | | | | ✓ | | |
| Body image | ✓ | ✓ | | ✓ | | | ✓ | ✓ | | ✓ | |
| Continence | | | | | | ✓ | | | | | ✓ |
| Facial swelling | | ✓ | | | | | | | | | |
| Fatigue | ✓ | | ✓ | | | ✓ | ✓ | | ✓ | | |
| Lymphoedema | ✓ | ✓ | | | | ✓ | | | | | |
| Muscle strength | ✓ | | | ✓ | | | | ✓ | | | |
| MSCC | ✓ | | | | | | ✓ | | | | ✓ |
| Nutritional problems | ✓ | ✓ | ✓ | ✓ | ✓ | | | | ✓ | | |
| Osteoporosis risk | ✓ | | | | | | | | | | ✓ |
| Pain | ✓ | ✓ | | | | | ✓ | | | | |
| Posture problems | ✓ | ✓ | | | | | ✓ | | | | |
| Radiation fibrosis | ✓ | ✓ | ✓ | | | | | | | | |
| Respiratory complications | | ✓ | ✓ | | | | | | | | |
| Scarring | ✓ | ✓ | | | | | | | | ✓ | |
| Sexual function | | | | | | ✓ | | | | | ✓ |
| Shoulder dysfunction | ✓ | ✓ | | | | | | | | | |
| Stiffness | ✓ | ✓ | | | | | | | | | |

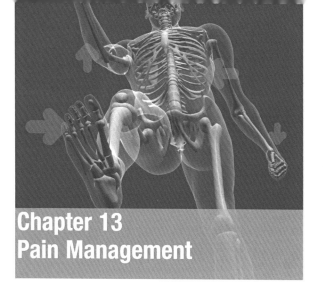

# Chapter 13
# Pain Management

## Introduction

Pain is a frequent part of everyday life with wide-ranging causes, e.g. unaccustomed activity/inactivity, bumps, bruises and indigestion, chronic disease or pain conditions. Pain may act as an acute internal warning, entering the consciousness insistently, or as a result of tissue damage.

Even premature babies have a fully functioning pain system and using morphine for their pain has a significant effect on morbidity and mortality. Heel stab and circumcision studies have demonstrated that the experience of early pain has a profound impact on future pain response (Goldschneider 1998).

Pain as a symptom is defined by the International Association for the Study of Pain (IASP) as 'an unpleasant and emotional experience associated with actual or potential tissue damage, or described in terms of such damage' (Merskey 1979). This encourages us to view pain as a complex perceptual experience that involves sensory-discriminative, affective-motivational and cognitive-evaluative components and not merely sensory information (Melzack and Casey 1968).

Wall (1989) described pain as a 'need state' in the way that hunger is, rather than a pure nociceptive sensation. Hunger drives the urge to find food, with relief of hunger being related more to expectations of the effect of eating rather than directly related to actual blood sugar levels.

Similarly, pain drives the urge to:

1 Escape from its cause: verified by the involvement of the motor cortex and cerebellum in pain processing. Movement strongly influences these controls from both the periphery and the brain. Wall (1995) suggested that 'the input may be better perceived in terms of the motor action which is appropriate, so that sensory and motor control are seen as two sides of the same coin', and (Wall 1999a Epilogue) 'pain is not just a sensation but … is an awareness of an action plan to be rid of it.'

2 Seek relief: this is supported by the fact that pain intensity is reduced in the presence of an intervention perceived as adequately effective in dealing with the

cause, even if its actual therapeutic effect is zero (Wall 1999b). The placebo response can be powerful; the effect of sham surgery can last for 6 months or longer (Cobb et al 1959). Pain is the main driver for patients to present to health care establishments and the most frequent symptom encountered by health professionals.

## Is the pain acute or chronic? Is there a difference?

Understanding pain as merely a signal of damage has hampered clinicians' and patients' views about how pain should be managed; clinicians and patients need to rethink what acute and chronic pain are. Moseley and colleagues have demonstrated that understanding what pain is has a significant real effect upon pain intensity and disability (Moseley et al, 2004).

### Acute pain

Acute pain is defined as pain that occurs at the time and for a period following injury, disease process or acute ischaemia. Signals from damaged tissue are relayed to the central nervous system (CNS) via nociceptors and nociceptive neurons (Woolf and Ma 2004).

Upon reaching the CNS, nociceptive signals may be automatically modified by factors that demand attention. These include the perceived threat of the situation and injury, past experiences, genetic factors, environmental and cultural factors, expectations and beliefs (Moseley 2007). Nociceptive signal reduction can be such that major injuries can, for a period, be experienced as pain-free, allowing for defensive and escape behaviours (Fanselow and Sigmundi 1986, Wall 1999a Chapter 1). Some minor injuries though can seem disproportionately painful. The CNS, therefore, does not merely passively relay and receive information.

When acute conscious pain occurs it is also accompanied by widespread reactions: alertness, orientation, attention and exploration, changes to heart and breathing rates and blood pressure, sweating, slowing of gut motility and rising anxiety (Wall 1999a). This is not just to support 'flight and fight' but also to initiate seeking (appropriate) help. Acute pain then continues to quite a varying degree while the healing, autoimmune, ischaemic or infective inflammatory processes are on-going. Inflammatory processes or peripheral nerve damage produce further integration of the distinctive patterns of adaptive, neuronal changes in the CNS (Milan 1999). Changes in the thalamus and somatosensory cortex can lead to quite marked hypersensitivity, frequently mistaken for inflammation. Inflammation is usually fairly transitory, its limit for even major injuries being at most a week (Evans 1980). Such changes usually resolve when the nociceptive stimuli stop.

During this recovery period however, symptoms can still be aggravated by certain physical factors such as prolonged immobilisation at any stage, or over-use in the early stages. Emotional factors such as stress, anger, depression, anxiety and anticipation (Main et al 2008 Chapter 2) can also amplify symptoms; many areas of the brain involved in pain processing are also activated during the experience of emotions. Emotions of course will partly be driven by beliefs and expectations; something that physiotherapists can influence.

### Chronic pain

Chronic pain is defined as pain that continues past the expected healing time or on-going pain (IASP 1994). An arbitrary time-frame of 3 months post onset/injury is a practical cut-off point for confirming the diagnosis of chronic pain since primary healing of all injury types will have been completed by then. Minor injuries (cuts, minor fractures, sprains) will have healed much faster and signs of chronicity can sometimes be picked up soon after injury:

• Mirror pains appearing on the contralateral limb.
• Sharp, shooting or stabbing pain.
• Burning pain.
• Feelings of swelling, stiffness, hot/cold.
• Colour changes.
• Paraesthesia/numbness.
• Feelings of ants crawling/water flowing/feels woody, etc.
• All movements hurt (not in normal distribution).
• Unpredictable.
• Pain has a 'mind of its own'.
• Pain increases with weather changes.

Fifty per cent of those with chronic pain remember no causative factors as the brain has the ability to generate a perception of pain without a nociceptive input (Tracey 2005). Chronic pain is distinguished from acute pain by the involvement of the pain system producing on-going central sensitisation (Sterner and Gerdle 2004).

These symptoms may present with acute pain and nerve damage, but there is an obvious injury and these resolve quickly.

Some patients with central sensitisation pain can have on-going perceptual problems, e.g. a limb feeling swollen when it is not, or is difficult to determine where it is, including sense of left/right and problems with discrimination (Lotze and Moseley 2007; Moseley 2004). Since these features were not recognised in the past, patients may have been worried that their problem was more serious than their health professionals considered it to be.

## Episodic pain

Episodic (or recurrent) pain is a form of chronic pain. Many patients presenting with apparent acute low back pain (LBP), may be experiencing an episode of an on-going chronic problem which has not been precipitated by accidental damage. Much of the misunderstanding around 'damage' caused by lifting is due to poor knowledge about the strength of bones and ligaments, and what pain perception actually is: allodynia is a hypersensitivity state, not actual damage.

Physiotherapists will be aware of physical and lifestyle factors that can contribute to pain recurring without apparent injury: a stiff joint above/below, chronic muscle tension, post-immobilisation or inactivity, stress, depression, lack of refreshing sleep, smoking. However, all these states occur in pain-free individuals too, so their effect on individuals cannot be linked with absolute certainty. Central hypersensitivity is the common factor.

## Summary

Acute nociceptive pain will have a clear injury or disease-process cause, settling within the expected healing time. It requires assessment and treatment for the underlying cause, but also assessment and management of the pain sensation and those factors that increase its impact.

In chronic pain however, both patients and clinicians should realise that the main focus for assessing, understanding and treating the pain should be that it is primarily a problem of pain transmission and perception, i.e. a problem within the nervous system. The cause is not tissue-based any longer, whether or not the tissues were originally injured or have a role in the maintenance of the problem.

Many patients are mystified by their pain experience. Your assessment aids understanding, which will help them accept it as a normal response, understandable, and within their power to modify or cope with.

## Key risk factors for chronic pain disability

The roles of musculoskeletal tissues and lifestyle factors in continuing pain are uncertain. However, somewhat more certain are the risk factors that contribute to chronic pain disability.

Most people who experience post injury pain have little hesitation in gradually reintroducing movements and activities. They may seek some reassurance or advice, but they generally manage recovery and rehabilitation instinctively and reasonably well. This is not always the case however, and until recently, the incidence of chronic pain disability was rising exponentially. Chronic pain and disability prevention is thus as important for acute pain as acute pain treatment. The importance of psychosocial factors in the development of these chronic problems has consistently been demonstrated (Shaw et al 2005) (Box 13.1).

It is important to consider the presence of risk factors for chronic pain disability – yellow flags – in every individual with acute pain, and assess these more thoroughly if they are suspected. Interventions can then be used to reduce the risk of disability, return patients rapidly to their usual level of fitness, and reduce the chances of acute pain becoming chronic.

## Assessment for pain: different presentations, pain syndromes

Distinguishing acute nociceptive from chronic pain and assessing risk factors for chronic pain disability should be part of the standard assessment. Pain has different presentations, and requires assessment to distinguish the type of pain or pain syndrome. This will allow you to inform your patients of the known and unknown aetiology of their condition and provide appropriate intervention. It will ensure you avoid unhelpful advice and treatment which may lead patients to think that their problem is serious or unmanageable.

---

**Box 13.1** Early risk factors for chronic pain disability (adapted from Shaw et al 2005)

- Patients with increased pain affecting sleep despite analgesia
- Belief that pain is harmful or potentially disabling
- Fear avoidance behaviour from fear of pain or fear of harm/causing damage
- Catastrophising (thinking the worst)
- Low mood due to pain and the consequences of injury
- Expectation that passive treatments rather than active participation in therapy would help
- Patients not making expected improvements 2–4 weeks after treatment for an acute (LBP) problem
- Patients who have significant difficulty with ADL or work, for more than 4 weeks (there is evidence for this factor for LBP and whiplash-associated disorders, but look for it with any pain)

The IASP have produced referenced clinical updates on each of these pain syndromes (http://www.iasp-pain.org).

## Neurogenic pain: slowly developing regional musculoskeletal or 'neuralgia-like' pains

These pains classically have no obvious causative injury. A period of unaccustomed work or activity may precede it, but recovery with paced activity would normally be expected to occur, but does not. A poor tolerance for static positions, for activity and/or stress of the body region, and reduced fitness of the whole body or body region ensues. Examples include syndromes such as repetitive strain disorder, epicondylitis, LBP and osteoarthritic pains which are becoming recognised as neurogenic pains and not tissue-based conditions (e.g. Laursen et al 2006). Comparing X-ray changes with normal subjects of similar ages shows little difference apart from pain hypersensitivity. Clear fMRI evidence is emerging of changes in the sensory cortex (Flor et al 1997). Neurogenic pain is not limited to the musculoskeletal system: some pelvic and bladder pains, chronic indigestion, irritable bowel and headaches are all now considered to be neurogenic pain. Such cases are often referred to non-pain specialists where focus on the painful tissues often leads to a poor outcome.

## Neurogenic pain: chronic widespread pain and fibromyalgia syndrome (FMS)

FMS is a non-articular disorder of unclear aetiology characterised by widespread pain throughout the body. The commonly encountered features of FMS are listed in Box 13.2.

There are few long-term studies and none with disease controls, so findings cannot be verified as specific to FMS. Evidence is growing for genetic, environmental and lifestyle factors (e.g. obesity, reduced fitness and poor sleep) affecting susceptibility.

External events including trauma, a regional pain syndrome, psychological distress, emotional trauma or an acute illness may trigger these pains. Among psychosocial stressors, the workplace has been found to be a main contributor.

Recent FMS criteria proposed by the American College of Rheumatology (Wolfe 2010) introduced a 'Widespread Pain Index' and a 'Symptom Severity Score.' Clinical relevance however remains to be explored.

---

**Box 13.2** Frequently reported features of fibromyalgia

- Widespread musculoskeletal pain, typically diffuse or multifocal
- Morning stiffness
- Joints or limbs feel swollen
- Headaches
- Temporomandibular joint dysfunction
- Irritable bowel syndrome; bladder disturbances; dysmenorrhoea
- Fatigue, reduced energy and drive
- Disturbed sleep; non-restorative sleep
- Problems with concentration, attention, or memory
- Mood disturbance

---

## Neuropathic pain

This is spontaneous pain and hypersensitivity associated with primary injury or dysfunction of the nervous system following peripheral nerve or spinal cord trauma or where disease process has damaged peripheral nerves, e.g. shingles, diabetes, human immunodeficiency virus (HIV)/acquired immune deficiency syndrome, alcoholism, vasculitis and multiple sclerosis. Following stroke, spinal cord injury or syringomyelia, patients frequently develop neuropathic pain. Changes occur in peripheral afferents, causing ectopic discharges at the site of the injury, at any neuromas and at the dorsal root ganglion (Woolf 2004).

Self report questionnaires have been developed to evaluate the presence of neuropathic pain such as 'painDETECT' which was developed to assess the neuropathic components of LBP (Freynhagen et al 2006) and the Leeds Assessment of Neuropathic Symptoms and Signs (LANSS) (Bennett 2001).

## Chronic regional pain syndrome (CRPS)

CRPS begins as rapidly escalating post-injury pain. Genetic factors have been identified that predispose to the development of CRPS. The extent of mechanical hyperalgesia in CRPS has been correlated to the extent of cortical reorganisation assessed on fMRI (Pleger et al 2006).

There are two types of CRPS, both ranging from moderate to extremely severe pain, each with different causes:

- CRPS type I: following minor injuries or fracture of a limb.
- CRPS type II: following injury to a major peripheral nerve.

Reluctance to reduce protective behaviour or to move unless the pain is reduced, can quickly lead to a cycle of avoidance, increased pain, demands for help, increased fear of painful movements, muscle tension in many areas, and fear of the future.

Stiffness, on-going spasm and signs of developing CRPS emerge.

Recognition of early stage CRPS may follow the removal of a cast, e.g. post Colles fracture, where the patient holds the now healed wrist as if it is still fractured. The Budapest criteria can provide a helpful framework for defining a diagnosis of CRPS (Box 13.3).

Quantitative sensory testing can be performed using von Frey hairs or Semmes–Weinstein filaments to assess whole body tactile thresholds and the extent of the allodynia, since some patients with CRPS develop contralateral or widespread remote symptoms (http://www.ugobasile.com/media/catalogue/products/leaflets/37450-277-von-frey-hairs-leaflet.pdf).

## Subjective assessment

Unlike a temperature, rash or a broken leg, pain can't be seen or tested for, it is a subjective, personal experience. Clinicians, carers and family should be alert to the possible presence of pain and clinicians should have the skills and tools necessary to systematically assess pain, which has been referred to as 'The Fifth Vital Sign™' (http://www.ampainsoc.org/whatsnew/painmonth05/downloads/FactSheet.pdf).

When pain is present, a detailed pain history should be taken including assessment of the multidimensional aspects of pain:

- A sensory dimension (the intensity, site and nature of pain).
- An affective/evaluative dimension (the emotional component of pain and how pain is perceived, e.g. dangerous, exhausting, frustrating, frightening).
- Impact on life, including physical, functional and psychosocial effects.

> **Box 13.3** Budapest Clinical Diagnostic Criteria for CRPS (Harden et al 2010)
>
> 1 Continuing pain, which is disproportionate to any inciting event
>
> 2 Must report at least one symptom in three of the four following categories:
>
> - Sensory: reports of hyperaesthesia and/or allodynia
> - Vasomotor: reports of temperature asymmetry and/or skin color changes and/or skin color asymmetry
> - Sudomotor/oedema: reports of oedema and/or sweating changes and/or sweating asymmctry
> - Motor/trophic: reports of decreased range of motion and/or motor dysfunction (weakness, tremor, dystonia) and/or trophic changes (hair, nail, skin)
>
> 3 Must display at least one sign at time of evaluation in two or more of the following categories:
>
> - Sensory: evidence of hyperalgesia (to pinprick) and/or allodynia (to light touch and/or deep somatic pressure and/or joint movement)
> - Vasomotor: evidence of temperature asymmetry and/or skin color changes and/or asymmetry
> - Sudomotor/oedema: evidence of oedema and/or sweating changes and/or sweating asymmetry
> - Motor/trophic: evidence of decreased range of motion and/or motor dysfunction (weakness, tremor, dystonia) and/or trophic changes (hair, nail, skin)
>
> 4 There is no other diagnosis that better explains the signs and symptoms

*This box has been reproduced with permission of the International Association for the Study of Pain ® (IASP®). The information may not be reproduced for any other purpose without permission.*

## Sensory dimension: pain intensity

- According to Labus et al (2003) the correlation between intensity and pain behaviour, intensity and disability is weak, therefore, why measure pain?

   *We must acknowledge patients' pain. Asking them to rate the intensity of their symptoms is a complex but important part of the assessment process.*

### The Visual Analogue Scale (VAS) and Numerical Rating Scale (NRS)

Patients can indicate the intensity of their pain on a 10 cm line (VAS) or choose a number from 0 to 10 (NRS). The NRS is easy to teach patients, and unlike the VAS, can be administered verbally, even by telephone (Figure 13.1a, b).

These apparently simple ratings of pain by patients actually incorporate a wide range of factors (Williams et al 2000) but have the advantage of being repeatable and easily systematised.

For young children between 3 and 7 years or those with learning difficulties the FACES pain rating scale can be used (Figure 13.2).

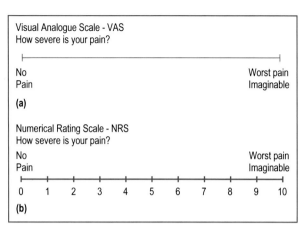

**Figure 13.1** (a) Visual analogue scale. (b) Numerical rating scale.

For some patient groups it can be difficult or impossible to speak about their pain and some psychological states or diseases can seriously affect communication. Time is required to recognise and interpret non-verbal expressions of pain for these more vulnerable members of society. Details of such tools can be found in Powell et al (2010).

### Sensory dimension: pain site

For musculoskeletal management, body diagrams are completed more comprehensively and precisely than for medical consultations, ensuring all pain/s and any other sensations of the whole body are included (Figure 13.3). Patients try to judge what we want and may fail to mention information if it is not specifically asked for, e.g. 'I'm here for my back, not my knee', 'My wrist pain is just from using my crutch'.

Closed questions produce poor data: 'Do you get headaches?' is less effective than 'Where do you have a headache when you get one?' then 'How often do you get a headache?'

### Sensory dimension: pain nature

The nature, quality and changeability of pain should be determined. Do not be surprised about some of the strange descriptions patients give you. What they tell helps to understand their predicament and highlights the remarkable things (lies even!) our brain can tell us.

Patients who feel water trickling down their leg, insects crawling under the skin or whose foot feels huge even when it clearly is not may have wondered if they are going mad. Fascination is a much more useful response from physiotherapists than disbelief. Obtaining details of sensation and perception have made us realise these are altered in a significant proportion of patients and that central sensitisation is behind most of our previous tissue-based diagnoses.

The McGill Pain Questionnaire (Melzack and Torgerson 1971) considers pain quality, but is not as diagnostic as originally hoped nor as useful clinically as asking the patient. It is no longer considered clinically relevant.

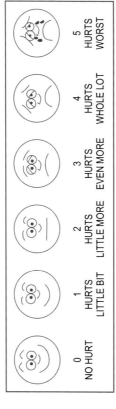

**Figure 13.2** FACES pain rating scale.

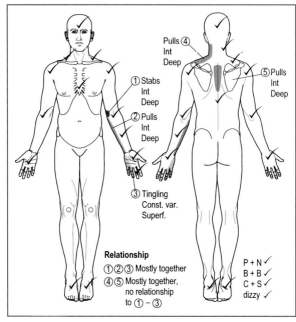

**Figure 13.3** Example of a completed body diagram. *Reprinted from Hengeveld E, Banks K 2005 Maitland's peripheral manipulation, published by Butterworth Heinemann, with permission of Elsevier Ltd.*

## Pain history

Basic patient demographic details and medical, pain and injury history need collecting, along with questions eliminating red flags.

Other subjective factors to document include:

- Usual activity at home, work, social/recreational interests and sport: what has stopped over the last year or so?
- Easing/aggravating factors; avoided activities or postures; sleep.
- Beliefs: why patients believe the pain started, why it is continuing and their understanding of pain mechanisms.
- Impact on patients' lives: losses in the realm of work or education, ADL, social and family life, and emotional distress.

Patients need to 'tell their story' during the assessment giving them opportunity to communicate with us. Many patients will have developed an explanatory model sometimes consisting of quite serious or worrying medical conditions or tissue damage and having a powerful effect on disability and quality of life. The story needs to be elicited and documented.

Allowing patients time to tell it in their way may save time! Key issues and concerns are more likely to emerge and, since patients sense when their information and their perspective is not fully respected, this is an important part of history-taking.

Few patients spontaneously disclose their ideas, concerns, and expectations. Often they suggest or imply their ideas through 'clues'.

Active listening is a skill for recognising and exploring these and will provide an enhanced understanding of patients' situations. Empathy and patience help build the therapeutic alliance.

Eye contact, actively indicating through body language that you have heard and are trying to understand, then summarising, will enable patients to correct any misunderstandings and give you insight into what is being conveyed both factually and emotionally. Nodding or saying phrases like 'I understand' or 'I see' shows acceptance, even if not necessarily agreement with patients' own theories. Unhelpful ones can then be a focus for change.

## Neuromusculoskeletal and physical function assessment

Establishing where pain is from and what it is affecting is essential. Physiotherapists can assess the local neuromusculoskeletal systems and the patient holistically. Appropriate clinical reasoning combined with experience will encourage a wider view of patients' problems and enable a clear focus on the key factors.

### Objective neuromusculoskeletal assessment

All patients should be assessed with appropriate outer clothes removed; it is possible to miss important signs if this is not done.

Gain consent and view different areas in stages, where possible, to maintain the patient's dignity. Chaperoning (not patients' family or friends) may be required to protect the clinician or at the request of the patient.

Key features for pain patients can include:

- *Skin*: signs of circulatory change, sympathetic nervous system activity, chronic tension and skin binding or freedom, abuse/harm, scars, acute/chronic swelling/oedema, avoidance of touch or pressure.
- *Posture*: reluctance with weight-bearing in standing or sitting; spine changes and right–left symmetry; effect of stiff joints, soft tissue tightness and muscle tension.
- *Range of movement*: general and specific. Hyper/hypoflexibility.
- *Strength*: consider muscle bulk, function and general movement; specific testing to assess neurological integrity; quality of muscle work, including muscle tone and muscle control.
- *Gait*: different surfaces, distances, speeds include stairs, squatting, 1-leg stance, lifting or carrying if appropriate.
- *Palpation*: Some pain states may preclude this, these patients may be able to give sufficient information about tenderness or skin quality themselves, or guide the palpation.

### Physical function

Evaluation of the impact of pain on patients' ability to maintain an independent functional lifestyle will indicate the risk of chronicity, the degree of fear avoidance behaviour and influence the physiotherapist's goals (which may be different from patients' goals).

## Patient self-report of physical function

Questionnaires can provide a quick assessment of the general degree of functional disability. This is useful for discussing patients with others, e.g. in case conferences, or when auditing outcomes. The choice of questionnaire(s) should take into consideration the department's patient population, why they are needed and what other centres are using, e.g. Roland and Morris Questionnaire for low back pain. Peat (2004) provides good advice on how to determine the merits and disadvantages of questionnaires and their use in clinical, audit or research settings.

Other tools include the Pain Disability Questionnaire, validated for chronic pain (Anagnostis et al 2004), Disabilities of the Arm, Shoulder and Hand (DASH) (Hudak et al 1996) and the Knee injury and Osteoarthritis Outcome Score (KOOS) (Roos et al 1998).

## Objective tests of physical function

It is not practical for a physiotherapist to assess all body areas. Effective observation of a specific range of functions will help focus objective assessment. Specific tools or techniques requiring little more equipment than a stop watch will provide objective evidence:

- 5-minute walk, 1-minute stair climbing, 1-minute stand-ups are part of a larger group of physical function measures developed for tertiary pain management programmes, but can also be used in outpatient primary and secondary care programmes (Harding et al 1994).

- Moores and Watson (2004) went on to develop this concept to concurrently and systematically assess physical pain behaviours.

- Clarke and Eccleston (2009) developed the 'Bath Assessment of Walking Inventory' a measure of the quality of walking in the presence of pain, for clinical and research use.

- Simmonds and colleagues developed physical function tests including the 5-minute walk, 50-foot speed walk, 5 repetitions of a sit-to-stand and loaded forward reach for patients with different conditions, e.g. LBP (Novy et al 2002), cancer (Simmonds 2002), HIV (Simmonds et al 2005) and lymphoma (Lee et al 2003).

- The Shuttle Walk Test (SWT) provides a greater challenge for patients than the 5-minute walk test, but requires equipment to provide a regular bleep sound and 2 traffic cones for patients to walk around (Singh et al 1992).

In pain patients these measures of function are more valid, reliable and responsive than traditional ROM and strength measures. They are meaningful outcome measures for patients and their referrers. The use of video means they can also be valuable clinical tools.

## Affective/evaluative dimension

### Depression

Since injury and pain can have a significant impact on a person's life (e.g. ability to engage in family life, work, social activities) low mood or depression are almost inevitable. Depression due to pain is itself linked to a higher risk of pain chronicity and can become a significant concern. To identify patients at risk, many departments now routinely administer the Depression, Anxiety, and Positive Outlook Scale (DAPOS) (Pincus et al 2008) or Hospital Anxiety and Depression Scale (HAD) (Snaith 2003). The physiotherapist should be familiar with these and when scores identify a problem requiring further evaluation, onward referral or urgent attention.

Departments that regularly see chronic pain patients may screen for depression using the Beck Depression Inventory (BDI) (Beck et al 1988) or short-form BDI (Steer et al 1999). Both are primarily screening tools to assess risk of suicide or self-harm and therefore should only be administered if there is direct access to psychological help if suicidal ideation emerges.

Many chronic pain patients have suicidal thoughts. Consult local guidelines and departmental protocols for working with suicidal patients: learn to recognise the signs and how to discuss these with such patients to ensure they know what to do to keep themselves safe.

## Anger and frustration

Assessment may reveal anger and/or frustration that may be focused on:

- The cause of the pain if the person feels powerless to have prevented it:
- An accident where someone else was at fault.
- Surgery or other intervention with a less than ideal outcome.
- The inadequacies of the Health System: they have not felt believed or taken seriously.
- Legal and medical assessments undergone for 'the other side', where their integrity has been questioned; where surveillance has been used to 'catch them out'.

Patients may need someone to listen in a non-judgemental way, believe them, explain the likely reasoning for decisions made, and suggest what can be done to help them move forwards.

It is rare, if this approach is taken, for anger to continue to be expressed in a way that feels disconcerting. If a patient continues to make you feel unsafe then this should be reported to a senior team member. A decision will need to be made for onward referral specifically for anger management or alternative strategies.

## Pain self-efficacy

Developed out of Bandura's (1977) work on self-efficacy, pain self-efficacy is the confidence to do things despite having pain. All voluntary behaviour change is regulated by self-efficacy. Patients with high self-efficacy are more likely to engage in coping behaviours because success is anticipated and they believe they can do them despite the pain (that is to say 'with it'). Patients with low levels however are less likely to use adaptive or helpful coping behaviours, believing that these may not be effective, or possible, in the presence of pain (Williams and Keefe 1991).

Patients understand self-efficacy as confidence. When a patient says 'I feel safe to walk without my stick here, but I couldn't go to the shops without my husband and my stick', and she has a wish to go shopping alone, then it can be identified that it is confidence that needs working on. Phrases like 'If I thought I wouldn't fall I'd do … xyz', 'I don't know if I can manage', 'I don't dare …' or indications that patients feel fragile, mean confidence is an important factor. Patients generally recognise its important role and the good feeling it brings, and usually wish to work on building it.

It is formally assessed using the Pain Self-Efficacy Questionnaire (PSEQ) (Nicholas 2007) which has been used in numerous studies by physiotherapists. It is reported as clinically very useful since this psychological construct is highly correlated with objectively measured physical function, is sensitive to change and an important predictor of pain management, physiotherapy outcome and return to work (RTW) (Tonkin 2008).

## Fear of movement (kinesiophobia)

Fear of movement, certain functions or situations that have become linked to pain or its onset, have an impact on physical function or work that is different to self-efficacy, although there is significant overlap (Kori et al 1990). The Tampa Scale for Kinesiophobia (TSK) is used quite widely in pain management and physiotherapy departments where graded exposure is being used for avoidance of movement due to fear (Clark et al 1996, Vlaeyen et al 2002). This can be useful to flag up those patients who have generalised fear-avoidance that requires a different approach to the usual exercise and activity pacing.

## Catastrophising

- Pain catastrophising, where patients view things in an overly negative way has been found to be consistently predictive of outcome. Patients reporting high levels of pain catastrophising also report higher levels of pain, psychological distress, and physical disability. High levels predict both future levels of pain and resulting disability.

- Catastrophising in these patients is best assessed using the Pain Catastrophising Scale (PCS) (Sullivan et al 1995, Keefe et al 2009).

- Catastrophising is not easy to change, so when significantly present seek assistance from a pain specialist physiotherapist or psychologist as the patient could need psychological intervention.

## Assessment of different patient groups

Guidelines are available for assessing pain in various patient groups including babies and the elderly (http://www.britishpainsociety.org/pub_professional.htm). Accident and emergency, intensive care, ward-based, outpatient departments and primary care centres will have their own guidelines for the assessment of pain.

## Assessing risk of chronic pain disability

Factors indicating a high risk of pain chronicity and disability can be seen soon after onset. Referred to as 'yellow flags' (Kendall et al 1997), the psychological risk factors for chronic pain disability are distinct from the red flag serious medical risk factors. The 'Acute Low Back Pain Screening Questionnaire' developed by Linton and Halldén (1998) was used to assess yellow flag risk indicators in LBP patients. The identification of risk factors for LBP chronicity and guidelines for management have been covered in detail by Van Tulder et al (2005), Main et al (2008) and Kendall et al (2009). The 'yellow flag' approach is now widespread; used routinely or when yellow flags are suspected. It ensures patients receive appropriate management from the onset (Watson and Kendall 2000).

This framework was further developed once the importance of workplace factors was established. Identification of relevant obstacles that delay recovery and RTW is now divided into three types (Main et al 2008, Kendall et al 2009):

- Yellow flags (about the person) – mainly psychosocial factors associated with unfavourable clinical outcomes and the transition to persistent pain and disability.

- Blue flags (about the workplace) from perceptions about the relationship between work and health, associated with reduced ability to work and prolonged absence.

- Black flags (about the context in which the person functions) include relevant people, systems and policies. These may operate at a societal level, or in the workplace and may block the helpful actions of healthcare and the workplace. Unchangeable factors need identifying so they can be navigated around. Black flags indicate the potential need to involve relevant others including professionals.

Remember the phrase: 'Person, Workplace, Context'. It emphasises appreciation of an obstacle, so it can be overcome or bypassed.

As with yellow flags, the blue and black flags do not necessarily indicate the presence or severity of persisting pain.

The references for this chapter can be found on www.expertconsult.com.

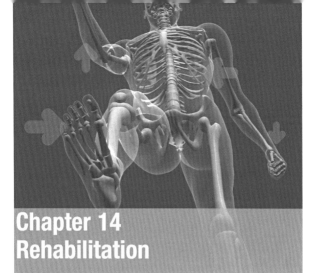

# Chapter 14
# Rehabilitation

## Introduction

*Rehabilitation is a combination of the processes of treatment and education that help disabled individuals to attain maximum function, a sense of well-being, and a personally satisfying level of independence.*

*Rehabilitation may be necessitated by any disease or injury that causes mental or physical impairment serious enough to result in functional limitation or Disability (Venes 2001).*

The fundamental principles that underpin rehabilitation in any health setting include:

- Assessment and evaluation
- Patient-centred care
- Goal setting
- Multidisciplinary team work.

## International Classification of Functioning, Disability and Health (ICF)

ICF is a useful framework for rehabilitation assessment that helps ensure that these principles are followed (WHO 2001).

The ICF represents a classification system of functioning, disability and health that can be used in any setting for any person. It provides a framework for rehabilitation assessments and management plans.

### Part 1

**Body functions**
The physiological functions of the body systems (including psychological, emotional, cognitive and physical functions).

### Body structures
Anatomical parts of the body such as organs, limbs and their components.

### Impairments
Problems in body function and structures, such as significant deviation or loss.

### Activity
The execution of a task or action by an individual.

### Participation
Involvement in a life situation.

### Activity limitations
Difficulties an individual may have executing activities.

### Participation restrictions
Problems an individual may experience in life situations.

## Part 2

### Environmental factors
The physical, social and attitudinal environment in which people live and conduct their lives. These are either barriers to or facilitators of the person's functioning.

### Personal factors
Age, sex, previous life experiences, personal choices and situations.

### Impairments
The older patient may have a number of impairments including weakness, pain, restrictions in range of movement, shortness of breath, pressure sores, incontinence, loss of proprioception, loss of memory, dysphasia and visual impairment.

Consider not only the physical impairments, but also the cognitive psychological and emotional functioning of the body. In clinical practice the individuals in a team of different professionals might take more interest in certain body structures and functions, e.g. physiotherapists will be most interested in the physical deviations, the occupational therapists in the cognitive functions and the psychologists in the emotional and psychological functions.

### Activity limitations and participation
Each profession should be aware of the impact of any impairment on the patient's ability to participate in activity. For example if the individual has weak muscles and is very anxious they might not be able to walk, therefore the activity limitation would be difficulty walking. The clinician should be aware of both the anxiety and the weakness as they may be impacting in equal measure on the activity limitation and participation restriction. Understanding the extent to which each type of impairment is impacting on the individual will allow the therapist to target their treatment plan for best effect. In the example if the anxiety has a greater impact than the weakness, the treatment should include confidence building and reassurance, in addition to strength training.

### Environmental and personal factors
The environmental factors make up the physical, social and attitudinal environment in which people live and conduct their lives.

The personal factors include peoples' attitudes, values and beliefs about their health, past and present experiences and how they perceive themselves. These are either barriers to or facilitators of the person's ability to function with a health condition. Being able to assess all these areas of the individual's presentation enables the practitioner to identify where his/her skills could help, where others might help and how to develop a customised care plan for the individual.

ICF is now used in health in various settings. It is recommended that rehabilitation therapists familiarise themselves with the ICF framework to help understand the individual's presentation from a holistic perspective (Sykes 2008).

## Fundamentals of the rehabilitation approach

### Assessment and evaluation

Assessment of the older person must include all the components of the ICF framework to allow the practitioner to consider the long-term impact of the acute presentation and be able to plan for their journey from an acute setting to their preferred destination which may be home or another community-based setting.

Following assessment the practitioner must consider how they will evaluate what they are doing.

Selecting an appropriate outcome measure will depend on what you are aiming to influence with your treatment programme. This may seem obvious, but often people choose an outcome measure that will not be sensitive to change and is not measuring what they want it to measure. For example global measures of functional change such as the functional independence measure (Stineman et al 1996) or the Rivermead motor assessment scale (Collen et al 1991, Lincoln and Leadbitter 1979, Sackley and Lincoln 1990) may not pick up changes in specific ranges of movement, whereas if you are working on outdoor mobility then the Community Mobility Index would be appropriate. Choose the right outcome measure to evaluate each individual's specific programme.

A helpful tip when looking at the outcome measures is to ask yourself which component of the ICF classification system is the measure focusing on, e.g. a visual analogue scale (VAS) (McCormack et al (1988)) could focus on any of the components, a pain VAS would be targeting the impairment, whereas a VAS on how easy it is to walk to the shops would be targeting the activity and participation component. Evaluation of interventions should not only consider objective measurement.

Today's practitioners should consider how to evaluate the patient experience and the use of patient-related outcome measures should be encouraged. Consider both the quantitative and qualitative evaluation of rehabilitation.

### Patient-centred care

It has been identified that practitioners sometimes fail to identify the patients' problems in a way that is meaningful to the patient. It is important that the clinician listens carefully to what the patient has to say during the assessment. It may take more than one session to collect all the information required. If the individual has difficulty communicating it may be necessary to collect information from other sources such as; carers, the patient's GP, relatives and friends, social services, previous medical records, reports from other disciplines are all sources of information which help build a picture of the individual. Failure to assess the environmental and personal aspects of the individual will make it difficult to identify what is important to the individual. Often the focus of the assessment is limited to the impairments of the body structure and function and how this impacts on the activity limitations. How these limitations impact on the individual's participation is vital. For example, if we take an older person who has been admitted from a nursing home with a chest infection and has previously been receiving full care and an older person who has been living with their family and enjoying full independent living. Both patients have the same impairment of admission with a chest infection, but the impact on their activities and participation is very different. Literature suggests that practitioners impose their views and opinions on the individual and do not work in partnership with their patients, to formulate a treatment plan that is patient-centred (Farin 2009). Recent publications suggest that there is a mismatch of views and poor listening skills amongst clinicians (Bloom et al 2006). Good patient-centred care relies on good communication skills, in particular listening (Reynolds 2004).

## Goal setting

Set goals from the patient's viewpoint. Goals need to be; specific, measurable, achievable, realistic and timed (SMART) (Bovend'Eerdt et al 2009). Goal setting can be a powerful motivator for patients, equally if the goal is too difficult it can have the opposite effect. Success is important to motivate patients.

Goal setting requires imagination and sensitivity, if the goal appears to be too difficult it is important to work with the individual to reset the targets to enable the goal to be achieved later. An example of setting appropriate goals may involve a patient that wishes to go home from hospital, what they need to do to achieve this is identified. This may involve the patient being able to roll to sit on the edge of the bed. This initial goal is then built upon by further goals working towards the ultimate goal of going home. The process is termed short- or long-term goal setting. The goals may be started in hospital, progressed into a rehabilitation setting either as an inpatient, outpatient, or indeed in the patient's own home. It is important to remember that anywhere along the pathway the practitioner needs to be able to help the person identify where they are going and how they will get there by re-evaluating the goals.

Goals can be anything your patient wants them to be, it is the therapist working with the patient that ensures that they are SMART.

Therapists sometimes find it difficult to set goals, due to the patient not being able to communicate their wishes, as a result of their impairments. In these cases the aim of the rehabilitation may be to manage the patient to get the optimal comfort, care and education goals can be set rather than functional goals.

The concept of active goals and passive goals has been used in the management of spasticity, these may be helpful in other areas (Richardson 1998). An active goal suggests that the patient will be performing some part of that goal themselves, e.g. to open and close the hand around a cup. An example of a passive goal is where the patient's carer opens the hand to cut and clean the nails. Both are achievable and patient-centred, but one involves active involvement and the other involves a carer achieving a care task. Active and passive goals can be patient-centred and SMART.

## Team work

It is important to remember that there is no 'I' in 'team', and that the patient is also part of the team. The ICF classification of function can assist a single assessor to identify other team members that might be of assistance. Team work requires good clear communication between the members and an understanding of each other's roles. Being able to identify where other team members' skills and knowledge could benefit an individual is a key part of the rehabilitation process (Nijius et al 2007, Shaw et al 2008). There are many specialist health services available for the care of patients that work together to effectively manage their problems. Consider a list of impairments for one individual and then think about the impact of these on activities and participation. Identify any contextual issues in the environment and the personal factors and then decide who would be the most effective team member to assist in meeting the needs of that individual. If we consider a frail older person who has fallen and is frightened of falling again, who also has a poor memory and does not go out very much, the impairments list might include, altered balance mechanisms, weakness in the legs, poor short-term memory, fear of falling, low mood. The activity limitations might be, unable to remember her tablets, frightened to go outside, social isolation. The team members that might be able to help could include the physiotherapist, the GP, the pharmacist, the voluntary visiting service, friends and family or neighbours.

## Assessment of the complex trauma patient

When confronted with a patient who has multiple injuries, the assessment, management and treatment can be quite daunting. But, by using a step-by-step approach and sound clinical reasoning, success is well within the reach of the student or junior clinician.

Patients who have been involved in serious trauma tend to have multiple problems. These include the physical, psychological and emotional as well as practical and vocational issues to be faced in the future. Because of this it is essential to take a holistic approach to patient care using all the resources of the multidisciplinary team (MDT).

On first contact it is useful to work through a general list of what you 'must do' in your assessment, as in any other. From this basic assessment, together with the patient you can formulate a management plan (Table 14.1).

Complex trauma can be exactly that, complex. Patients have a multitude of problems, all in some way impacting on each other and affecting your ultimate measure, function. It is essential to deal with the patient in a holistic manner with full input and good communication with the MDT.

There are many different presentations of conditions following trauma. Rarely do patients fit into one single category (orthopaedic fracture) without crossover from another (burns and plastic surgery). However, there are certain things that should be considered when dealing with specific presentations.

| Table 14.1 Initial assessment checklist | |
|---|---|
| Physical | Musculoskeletal assessment (ROM, Power) |
| | Neurology (myotomes/dermatomes) |
| | Comorbidities and their management (bladder & bowel) |
| | Pain (controlled?) |
| | Past and possible future surgery (weight-bearing status) |
| | Sexual function (plus its affect on psychological/ emotional elements) |
| | Aids to mobility (crutches/wheelchair) |
| Psychological | Personality/mood (present & prior to trauma) |
| | Patients understanding of the situation's gravity |
| | Mild traumatic brain injury |
| Emotional | Family support |
| | Relationship status (partner, children) |
| | Lifestyle (present & prior to trauma) |
| | Age/stage of life/career |
| Function | Premorbid function |
| | Present function |
| | Predicted function |
| | Short- and long-term goals |

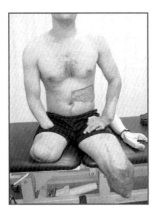

**Figure 14.1** Triple amputee, with extensive soft tissue injury.

## The amputee

Traumatic amputations can be simple (unilateral below knee) or complex (triple amputee) (Figure 14.1), but both have similar needs.

Assess the integrity (tissue) and functional ability (size, shape) of the stump. Close work with the prosthetic team is essential if mobilising on prosthetic limbs is a goal. They can advise on fitting/gait and prosthetic choice. The availability and development of prosthetic limb technology has progressed to such an extent that bilateral above-knee amputees can independently fully mobilise with no walking aids if rehabilitated correctly.

Rehabilitation should be underpinned by a good understanding of amputee biomechanics and gait analysis. The demographic of trauma patients is such that young previously fit men make up a large portion of the caseload and these individuals have and can achieve challenging goals and recover from a poorly conditioned status after endurance training (Chin et al 2002). Mountain climbing, paralympic competition and waterskiing can be realistic goals.

## Multiple fractures

With high-velocity road traffic accidents or indeed blast injuries from explosions there are often multiple injuries. It is not unusual to see a patient with pelvic, lower limb and spinal fractures. On presentation to you they will often have external fixation following surgery, with a number of further surgical interventions planned.

With these patients normal principles of assessment and treatment apply. A sound understanding of post op protocols (weight-bearing) and future plans is essential. Familiarise yourself with the surgical procedures and their objectives. There are often associated complications such as soft tissue trauma, malunion, compartment syndrome and infection (Figure 14.2). You should be looking to maintain and if possible improve available function as well as liaising with other members of the MDT regarding any complicating factors.

## Nerve and soft tissue damage

Patients with isolated soft tissue or nerve injuries are the exception rather than the rule. The velocity during trauma caused by a gunshot wound for example, is such that the two come hand in hand.

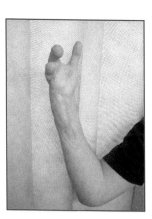

**Figure 14.2** Soft tissue injuries and associated bony disruption.

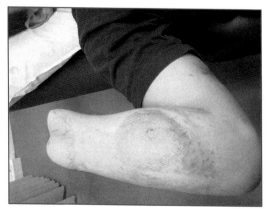

**Figure 14.3** Burn and graft site, upper limb.

A thorough knowledge and understanding of neural anatomy will help to ascertain what is causing weakness during function, deconditioning or structural damage to the nervous system. Patients may be hyper/hyposensitive in particular areas. It is essential to appreciate that nerve damage can lead to poor function of more than just the musculoskeletal system, e.g. bladder and bowel. Peripheral nerve injuries are common, but despite the fast advances in research and technology, a complete recovery following peripheral nerve injury is rare, however considerable progress has been achieved with the development of microsurgery techniques (Tuncali et al 2004).

Particular attention needs to be paid to the management of scar tissue to prevent contractures limiting movement. Patients often have associated burn and graft sites, which need attention (Figure 14.3). The patient needs to be convinced of the benefits of early management of soft tissue injuries in order to treat him- or herself and maximise long-term function.

## Psychological trauma

The psychological impact on patients involved in trauma must be considered at all times. The patient's life, and often the relationship between family and friends is changed forever. Some may initially appear euphoric and 'happy to be alive' only to psychologically 'crash' when the reality of future disability sinks in. Others will present with low mood, which can be lightened as progress is made.

Not all people who experience a potentially traumatic event will actually become psychologically traumatised (American Psychiatric Association 1994). Many people experience traumatic events during their life and it is normal to have strong feelings of anxiety, sadness, or stress. Some patients may even experience symptoms of what is known as post-traumatic stress disorder (PTSD) which may include night-mares, memories about the event, or difficulties sleeping (Storr et al 2007). Patients may be experiencing symptoms of PTSD, but only a mental health professional can confirm the diagnosis. Many of the symptoms of PTSD are part of the body's normal response to stress. An individual may experience an event as traumatic whereas another present at the same event may not feel any traumatic effect. Gaining an understanding of the patient's personality and nature pre and post trauma will help to monitor changes in mood and attitude during rehabilitation.

Communication within the MDT and referral to mental health professionals if required should form part of the treatment plan.

## Subjective information

Obtaining a detailed subjective history is essential for the formulation of an effective management plan. The patient is often the best source of information, but may not have any memories of the incident beyond the point of injury, e.g. following an explosion. In this case family members, the patients work mates/fellow soldiers or passengers in a vehicle may be helpful.

There will be medical notes from admission to hospital and surgical interventions and contributions from all members of the MDT. Reviewing these is important; as knowing about the success or failure of past interventions will aid future planning. If you are not the first physiotherapist to see the patient it is essential to receive a written or verbal handover for information.

In addition to the demographic subjective history further details are required to formulate a management plan (Table 14.2).

## Objective information

Keeping an objective record of treatments provided helps monitor progress and success. Power, range of motion and functional objective testing is a way to dem-onstrate meaningful progression and give both the therapist and patient confidence (Table 14.3).

## Treatment planning

Using the information from the subjective and objective assessment a reasoned treatment plan can be made. Despite the complex nature of some trauma every effort should be made to keep the plan simple. If a muscle group is weak and needs to be stronger, strengthen it.

A step-by-step approach thinking of what you must/should/could do will help the plan to take shape. Use achievable and measurable short- and long-term goals discussed with the patient to confirm progress and give positive feedback. Always remember physiotherapy for complex trauma need not be complex.

**Table 14.2** Trauma-specific questions

| Subjective information | Relevance |
|---|---|
| What was the trauma? Where did it happen? Who was involved? | Others may have been involved and possibly hurt |
| How does the patient feel about the incident? | Negative effect of psychological factors (PTSD) |
| Do they have emotional/financial/physical support? | Adequate support systems are essential to aid recovery |
| To what level do they expect to recover? | Realistic and attainable goals are essential |
| What career are they involved in? | May not be possible to return to that line of work |
| What interventions are already planned? | Further surgery will need to be accommodated |
| Is a family member/partner able to speak with you? | They may often provide a different perspective/view on patient's history |
| Do they have any dependants? | Partner or children may rely on them for financial support – can increase stress |

**Table 14.3** Outcome measures

| Testing tools | Reasoning | Testing tips |
|---|---|---|
| Amputee mobility predictor questionnaire (Gailey et al 2002) | Used early on during Ax to determine current (and potential) function, assists planning appropriate treatment and setting goals | A functional exercise programme can accompany the questionnaire providing guidance on treatment options |
| T – Test (Semenick 1990) | Simple and reproducible test of proprioception & balance/agility | The type of surface should be consistent to ensure reliability. A test for use with high-functioning patients |
| Multistage walk test/6Min walk test (ATS guidelines 2002) | The change in the distance walked in the 6MWT can be used to evaluate the efficacy of an exercise programme or to trace the natural history of change in exercise capacity over time | The MSFT can be employed for patients whose functional ability has progressed beyond the 6MWT. Standardisation of the six-minute walk test (6MWT) is very important |
| FIT HaNSA (MacDermid et al 2007) | Provides a brief measure of functional performance of the upper limb | Provides valid assessment of impaired functional performance in patients with shoulder pathology |

# Assessment of the musculoskeletal (sports) patient

The assessment of a patient following a musculoskeletal sports injury is carried out prior to rehabilitation and regularly during the rehabilitation process to ensure the patient is progressing appropriately. Without regular assessment the patient may receive daily treatment without meeting their goals within an appropriate timeframe. The process of assessment in musculoskeletal rehabilitation must be well organised with both subjective and objective assessment measures being used.

It is a common approach for some standardised tests to be carried, in order to collect some baseline data prior to rehabilitation starting. This often occurs when a patient has been injured or following an operation when they have been given a period of time to rest (in order to allow the injury to heal). Following a planned programme of rehabilitation the standardised tests would be repeated to ascertain the progress made by the patient. However, this two-point assessment approach often fails to enable the patient to achieve optimum recovery.

## The patient journey

The process of rehabilitation should be viewed as a journey along a road where there will be a series of roadblocks during the journey. At each roadblock, assessment and revision of the rehabilitation programme will be required until the end of the road is reached, i.e. full fitness is achieved. There are often guidelines to follow, set by a surgeon or specialist and also by our knowledge of the healing processes, biomechanics and physiology. To attain optimum healing during the rehabilitation process a certain tension must be applied to the healing tissues in the correct manner, at the appropriate level and at the right time, in order that 'windows of opportunity' are not missed. Regular assessment can help identify these windows and provide an indication about how far along the rehabilitation road the patient has travelled.

As an example: if guidance has been given by a specialist that the patient should not run for 6 months, your assessment will have to acknowledge this limitation. Therefore the plan should not include a goal that would aim to have the patient doing a 100-metre sprint test after 2 weeks. Following an injury to the posterior cruciate ligament in the knee, that has been identified as being a grade II injury, there will need to be a period of immobilisation for 6 weeks. The assessment must respect this, so that the window of opportunity for the ligament to heal at the appropriate length is not missed.

If a rigorous process of assessment is not followed then issues may arise.

The following example highlights where potential issues may arise during the rehabilitation period.

Following a rupture of the Achilles tendon, surgical repair and 6 weeks of immobilisation in a plaster cast the patient was told by the surgeon to walk at the 6-week postoperative check up. At this point the patient could not do so without difficulty, due to reduced range of movement, decreased strength and lack of confidence. The patient had met the time line for the surgeon; however, he had not met any of the essential criteria required for him to be able to walk normally. In any situation where there are changes in the permitted amount of weight bearing, e.g. from non-weight bearing to partial weight bearing, an assessment must be carried out as identified in Table 14.4.

As the example in Table 14.4 demonstrates, the rehabilitation of injuries such as these must be target led. The therapist must then ensure that the patient progresses to meet the targets. Again using the example of the patient following a rupture of

**Table 14.4** Example of progression from non-weight-bearing to partial weight-bearing gait

| Criteria | Goal | Assessment | Assessment findings | Treatment as Required | Re-assessment | Action | Target Full Weight-bearing |
|---|---|---|---|---|---|---|---|
| Ankle ROM | Achieve neutral DF | Goniometer to assess ankle ROM | Insufficient dorsiflexion | | Neutral DF achieved | Able to walk if other assessment criteria are met | |
| Muscle length tests | | Gastroc. and Soleus tests | Gastrocnemius tests tight | | Gastrocnemius = to other leg | | |
| Strength | Calf raise against gravity + some resistance | Oxford scale for muscle strength | Too weak to raise | | Standing calf raises | | |
| Balance | Both sides to be equal | a Joint position sense | R=L | | | | |
| | Both sides to be equal | b Double leg stance | R=L | | | | |
| | Both sides to be equal | c Single Leg stance | Unable to maintain | | R=L | | |

the Achilles tendon, it is the opinion of the surgeon that following removal of the cast the patient should commence walking when safely possible. The knowledge and experience of the therapist agrees with this.

## Targets

Targets are set in order for the patient to achieve a normal gait pattern. The criteria must be met and the goals achieved in order for the patient to meet the targets.

- Criterion 1. Muscle length → Goals → Assessment tools → Findings → Treatment → Assessment tools → Target reached
- Criterion 2. Muscle strength → Goals → Assessment tools→ Findings → Treatment → Assessment tools → Findings → Target reached

Criteria are prioritised with the most time consuming or the most demanding at the top. In criterion 1 the priority was identified as muscle length, the goal for this was to achieve neutral dorsiflexion. The assessment tool chosen to measure this was a goniometer, the findings were that the patient did not have neutral dorsiflexion. Treatment was carried out and the resulting increase in dorsiflexion to neutral dorsiflexion meant the patient was able to progress to full weight-bearing (FWB) gait. While the therapist was working to achieve the target for muscle length other criteria were addressed (criterion 2, muscle strength), with the goal being the ability to complete a single-leg calf raise. Strength was assessed using the Oxford grading system, the results show the calf is too weak to walk; therefore the patient is treated with exercises, in an aquatic therapy pool. Following reassessment the goal is achieved. This process is repeated for all criteria until the goals are attained and the target of FWB is achieved.

## Monitoring progression

To monitor the progression through the rolling roadblocks there are two assessment processes that are essential;

- Milestone assessment

  Used to measure milestone targets at certain key points during the rehabilitation process, e.g. when a patient moves from non weight bearing to partial weight bearing or from walking to running.

- Daily assessment

  Used on a daily basis to monitor the work level, intensity and load by using certain assessment criteria. This careful monitoring allows the rehabilitation to be progressive without aggravating the injury.

## Milestone targets and milestone assessment tools

For serious long-term injuries, such as an anterior cruciate ligament reconstruction, a ruptured Achilles tendon or post shoulder reconstruction five milestone targets are used, with the injury type dictating the timescale for each milestone.

The five main areas used are:

### Early assessment

After an initial injury or after surgery the aim is to create an environment to promote healing and to establish homeostasis. Gradual muscle activity is then introduced along with proprioceptive activity (Table 14.5).

Moving between milestones not all targets have to be met at the same time, some may progress quicker than others.

**Table 14.5** Early assessment milestones

| Area of rehabilitation | Assessment tools | Additional information | Targets | References |
|---|---|---|---|---|
| 1 Joint homeostasis | Measure joint circumference<br>Swelling tests<br>Heat | | Joint homeostasis | Magee (1997) |
| 2 Pain | Visual analogue scale | | | Magee (1997) |
| 3 Muscle strength | Manual testing | | Grade 2 or 3 mm power | Galley and Forster (1992) |
| | Baseline measurements of muscle girth | | | |
| 4 Muscle extensibility + joint range | Goniometer<br>Muscle length tests | This is very often a priority | Normal asap | Kendall et al (1993) |
| 5 Proprioception | Joint position sense | Can often be worked on early | Equal side to side | Herrington (2005) |
| 6 Gait | | Video analysis | | |
| 7 Anthropometric measures | Shin folds<br>Height<br>weight | | | |
| 8 Athletic measurements | Hypermobility screening | At this stage tests to monitor athletic performance to be used as base line measurements | | |
| | Musculoskeletal assessment | Leg length, spinal, hip mobility, box test, sij assessment | | |

### Mid assessment

The priority is to increase muscle strength, improve ROM and move the roadblocks further along the road to recovery. During this period the early phase must not be forgotten, as areas such as joint homeostasis must be monitored. At this stage as the workload increases the daily assessment tools become increasingly more specific and important (Table 14.6).

### Late assessment and functional assessment

This phase is where the aim of the patient can be considered more closely. Focus is on their job or the sport that they do (Table 14.7).

### Return to sport assessment

Returning a player to their sport is driven very much by the sport, injury, position and individual person. The therapist should have standardised tests with can be used as fitness tests at the final stage of rehabilitation before the individual is gradually reintroduced to the sport. For this to happen the functional tests in Table 14.7 must be equal side to side and must match preinjury data, particularly when a player has been out for a long time. Often a 10% deficit compared to preinjury data is considered to be acceptable, but this should be as low as possible before returning the patient to sport.

For lesser injuries such as a muscle strain or a strained ligament a similar process can be followed along the road to recovery, but less milestones may be necessary as the patient may progress quickly to the final target.

## Daily assessment tools

The daily assessment tools use both subjective questioning and objective testing. Questions such as: how were you on waking?, how is it now?, how much muscle soreness did you have on waking and how much now?, any swelling?, any pain? The answers can provide useful indicators of progression or deterioration. The objective tests may include; ROM, swelling, heat and gait observation. Together the subjective and objective findings are used to monitor and progress on a daily basis the work being carried out.

**Table 14.6** Mid assessment milestones

| Area of rehabilitation | Assessment tools | Additional information | Targets | References |
|---|---|---|---|---|
| 1 Joint homeostasis | Measure joint circumference<br>Swelling tests<br>Heat | | Joint homeostasis | Magee (1997) |
| 2 Balance tests | Walking<br>Lunge<br>Static hops | Observe load video analysis | Sides must be =<br>Good gait stairs | |
| 3 Strength tests | Sets and repetitions | 6 rep max etc. | | Baechle and Earle (2000) |
| 4 Functional tests | Core timed plank<br>Gluteal bridge<br>Squats<br>Vertical jump | These tests can be away from site of injury and can be tests that were used pre injury | Improve athleticism | |

**Table 14.7** Late assessment and functional assessment

| Area of rehabilitation | Assessment tools | Additional information | Targets | References |
|---|---|---|---|---|
| 1 Joint homeostasis | Continue to monitor | | | |
| 2 Joint range and muscle extensibility | | Normal or maximum should have been achieved | | Kendall et al (1993) |
| 3 Functional tests for strength, balance and co-ordination | Vertical jump | | | |
| | Functional movement screen | Can often be used throughout rehab | Pre-injury status | Ageberg et al (2008) |
| | Standing long jump | If you have preinjury data can be a very good indicator of readiness to return | | Wiklander and Lysholm (1987) |
| | Star excursion test | Very useful to compare sides | Sides = | Herrington et al (2009) Filipa et al (2010) |
| | 'Y' test | More simple than the star excursion test so can be used more often | | |
| | Cross over hop test | Very good dynamic test | | |
| | Static hop for distance | Good research on this test very useful if have preinjury data | | Pincivero et al (1997) Wilk et al (1994) |

## Traffic lights

A system that can assist daily assessment is the use of traffic lights with the colours being linked to the results of the subjective and objective assessment.

*Green* indicates that the previous day's work has not aggravated the joint or site of injury and the rehabilitation programme can continue and progress as planned.

*Red* indicates that the previous day's work or something that the patient has done has aggravated the area of concern and it means that action must be taken to retrieve the situation. This may involve stopping treatment and allowing the patient to have a complete day of rest, or if the findings are marked then a further clinical opinion may need to be sought. It is essential that the patient discloses anything that they may have done to aggravate the situation and at the very least something will need to be changed in the intervention plan to help the situation.

*Amber* involves the therapist making a decision about how to modify treatment. The decision will be based on clinical reasoning, drawing on evidence and clinical experience. It means that the previous day's activities have aggravated the area slightly and the therapist must decide what it was about these interventions that caused the aggravation and what to change. If the session the previous day was very demanding then the plan might be to reduce the repetitions, resistance or change the programme. However, if the session was relatively easy, then a more dramatic change may be needed, e.g. a day off, a pool day or a training day to work other areas of the body may be alternatives to be considered.

The system of traffic lights allows the clinician to monitor the workload and make subtle alterations as the process progresses. Using the analogy of driving along a straight road that has many sets of traffic lights, it is the experience of the author that if you encounter the first set of lights on red then you seem to hit them all on red, whereas if the first set of lights is green they all seem to be green and the journey is shorter and more pleasant. This seems to be the same for rehabilitation if in the early stages the daily assessments are green then the patient's journey seems to progress well. If red lights appear early in the patient's rehabilitation programme then this means that there may need to be more investigations to ascertain why the patient has failed to progress and the timeframes for progression are likely to be prolonged.

The frameworks included in this chapter can be used and adapted for all injuries that require a rehabilitation approach.

The references for this chapter can be found on www.expertconsult.com.

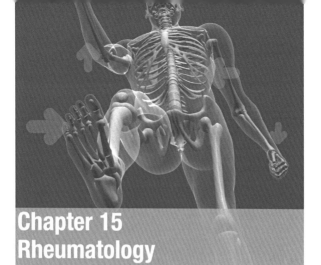

# Chapter 15
# Rheumatology

## Introduction

- Rheumatology covers a wide range of conditions affecting the musculoskeletal system including all types of arthropathies and soft tissue conditions such as tendonitis and bursitis.

- Also included are less common auto-immune conditions such as connective tissue disorders and vasculitis.

- Many long-term conditions can be managed by different specialist areas of physiotherapy.

- Chronic pain management may be managed by pain specialists in some geographical areas, whereas in others a rheumatology service will have the remit for managing chronic pain.

- Physiotherapy for rheumatological conditions is built upon the core skills that are used in all areas of musculoskeletal practice.

- This volume anticipates that the reader will possess a basic level of knowledge and experience of musculoskeletal assessment, i.e. that they will be able to carry out an assessment of joint range or muscle power.

- The material in the volume will guide the reader in how they may apply core skills in the assessment of patients with inflammatory arthritis.

## Current trends in management of inflammatory arthritis

- The medical treatment of inflammatory arthritis is a rapidly developing area of healthcare.

- In the recent past there have been major advances in drug treatment offering significant improvements in long-term function and disease management within inflammatory arthritis.

- Whereas in the past a physiotherapist would expect to see large numbers of patients with significant disability levels, these are now being encountered less frequently.
- Due to these changes the role of the rheumatology physiotherapist is sometimes poorly understood and appreciated within the profession.

## The purpose of assessment

### Identification of potential case of currently undiagnosed inflammatory arthritis

- Increasing numbers of patients are choosing to self-refer to physiotherapy. This means that physiotherapists can often be a first point of contact for a patient with an undiagnosed rheumatological condition (Cleland and Walter-Venzke 2003).
- Early diagnosis and treatment is the basis of modern rheumatology, any suspected cases of new inflammatory arthritis should be referred to specialist services.
- Box 15.1 outlines the National Institute for Health and Clinical Excellence (NICE) guidance for the early referral of suspected new cases of rheumatoid arthritis (NICE 2009).
- It is important to ask specific questions during the assessment which can help identify the presence of inflammatory back pain.
- It is worth noting that with inflammatory arthritis of peripheral joints or the axial skeleton there is no single definitive diagnostic test which can be used; diagnosis is achieved through a combination of examination, considering the features that the patient presents with (Box 15.2), history taking and the appropriate application of specific diagnostic tests and techniques.

### Assessment and diagnosis of inflammatory arthritis

- This will be significantly influenced by the involvement of other health professionals, the phase of drug treatment the patient is in, the disease process, and ultimately the patient's expectations and aspirations.
- Physiotherapists will invariably practice within a multidisciplinary team, usually comprised of:
- Medical staff
- Nurses
- Occupational therapists (OT)
- Dieticians
- Orthotists
- Podiatrists
- Psychologists
- Pharmacists (Luqmani et al 2009).

> **Box 15.1** Guidance for early referral of suspected cases of rheumatoid arthritis
>
> Refer for specialist opinion any person with suspected persistent synovitis of undetermined cause. Refer urgently if any of the following apply:
> - the small joints of the hands or feet are affected
> - more than one joint is affected
> - there has been a delay of 3 months or longer between onset of symptoms and seeking medical advice (NICE 2009)

> **Box 15.2** Features of inflammatory arthritis
>
> - Tender, warm, swollen joints
> - Symmetrical pattern of affected joints
> - Joint inflammation often affecting the feet, wrists and finger joints
> - Joint inflammation affecting other joints, including the neck, shoulders, elbows, hips, knees, ankles, and feet
> - Fatigue, occasional fevers, a general sense of not feeling well
> - Pain and stiffness lasting for more than 30 min in the morning or after a long rest
> - Symptoms that last for many years
> - Variability of symptoms among people with the disease (NIAMS 2009)

## Review assessment

- These tend to be undertaken as part of a regular planned review process of patients with rheumatoid arthritis and ankylosing spondylitis by a rheumatology team, in accordance with the NICE guidelines (NICE 2009).
- ASAS/EULAR recommend that the frequency of monitoring in ankylosing spondylitis (AS) should be decided for each individual patient based on symptoms and disease severity (Kiltz et al 2009).

## Triage assessment

- This is a developing area for physiotherapists working within a rheumatology team. Additional training in specific diagnostic and therapeutic skills has expanded the role of the rheumatology physiotherapist in a way that has been established in orthopaedics for a number of years (Weatherley and Hourigan 1998, Pearse et al 2006).

## Subjective assessment

- It is important to record information on a body chart (Figure 15.1). This provides a baseline of the patient's symptoms on the first attendance which should change in response to physiotherapy intervention.
- Central to the whole assessment process is the interaction between clinician and patient.
- At the beginning of an assessment it is essential to establish a rapport with the patient, provide explanations about what the assessment entails, and obtain their consent.

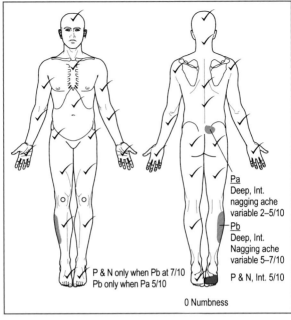

**Figure 15.1** Body chart for recording presence of a patient's symptoms.

- Consent is an ongoing, interactive process that will need to be sought throughout the assessment and subsequent treatment (CSP 2005).

## Patient-defined problems, health beliefs, expectations and mood

- Gaining an understanding of the impact of the condition on the patient's function and lifestyle is crucial to the therapeutic process.
- This will have a direct bearing on the short- and long-term physiotherapy interventions and the patient's undertaking of 'self management'.
- A general evaluation of mood can be useful to consider if a patient seems depressed or anxious.
- Use of validated measures such as the Hospital Anxiety and Depression Scale (HADS) may identify affected mood in appropriately selected patients (Zigmond and Snaith 1983).
- Function can be affected in inflammatory arthritis, causing some tasks to become difficult and others impossible (Table 15.1).
- A number of validated measures exist to evaluate this, for example the Health Activity Questionnaire (HAQ) (Fries et al 1980).
- At times it can also be useful to assess health-related quality of life using validated measures such as EQ5D (The EuroQoL Group 1990).

**Table 15.1** Potential functional impairments in rheumatological conditions

| Peripheral joints | Axial skeleton |
|---|---|
| Using a toilet, getting in or out of a bath | Getting out of bed in the morning |
| Washing hair, cleaning teeth | Putting socks on in morning |
| Dressing | Back stiffness after prolonged sitting |
| Climbing stairs | Back stiffness after prolonged standing |
| Walking, speed, distance and rhythm, on uneven or unstable surfaces | Reaching high cupboard or washing line |
| Household activities, e.g. Cooking | Lifting and carrying |
| Opening packets and jars | Rolling in bed |
| Picking up and using keys | Driving |
| Writing | Reversing when driving |
| Driving | Walking speed, distance and rhythm |
| Hobbies, e.g. knitting | |
| Care activities for others, e.g. dressing children | |
| Sports performance | |
| Paid employment | |

- Throughout the assessment it is necessary to consider how the various aspects of functional impairment relate to the underlying rheumatological condition and what is important to the patient.

- During any discussion of function it is important to identify how the skills of the physiotherapist may assist the patient with their functional activities and where other professions may have a role to play.

- Major functional limitation may entail referral to an occupational therapist. Good team communication and working is essential here.

## Pattern of joints affected by rheumatoid arthritis

- Inflammatory arthritis will typically develop a characteristic pattern of joint involvement.

- A rheumatology body chart can be used to record specific joint palpation finding (warmth, pain swelling).

- It can be useful to have larger hands because of the relatively high occurrence of arthritis in this area and therefore facilitate the recording of greater detail (Figure 15.2).

## Behaviour of signs and symptoms

### Swelling/temperature

- The pattern of painful and swollen joints in inflammatory arthritis can vary for the different types of arthritis.

- Given the often protracted nature of the problems before the assessment, patients can sometime lack precision in describing swelling and other features.

- A feature of the spondyloarthropathies is dactylitis (swelling of a whole digit), and in acute arthritis joints can appear warm.

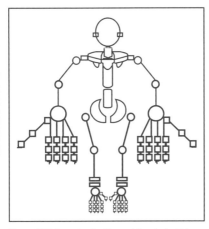

**Figure 15.2** Example of a Rheumatology bodychart.

Joint stiffness

- The stiffness associated with inflammatory arthritis is typically worse after periods of immobility.
- Significant times for this are getting out of bed in the morning, getting up after prolonged sitting and sustaining a fixed position.
- Morning stiffness of more than 30 minutes is an important diagnostic feature of inflammatory arthritis, but the stiffness duration can sometimes be shorter.
- In the context of discussing pain and stiffness it can often be helpful to take the patient through a typical day to allow them to highlight the variation in the symptom pattern, which in inflammatory arthritis will tend to be worse in the first half of the day.

Pain

- It is helpful to define the areas affected as precisely as possible. In arthritis the pain, stiffness and swelling often coincide within the same general area.
- In chronic rheumatological conditions pain may seem confusing because the patient may report pain associated with inflammation in a specific joint and also arising from secondary degenerative changes, other long-term but uninvolved conditions, or pain which might lack a specific physical cause.
- Noting the patient's description of pain can help to determine the structures involved, e.g. sharp and shooting may indicate nerve root involvement.
- Note the behaviour of the pain in response to movement and activity, also the patient's beliefs about their symptoms.
- Patients may also report pain and swelling at the entheses (the insertion of tendons into bone), known as enthesitis. If a spondyloarthropathy is suspected or diagnosed there is the possibility of enthesitis occurring (Colbert 2010). This can be assessed by careful palpation and using an enthesitis index Appendix 15.1. Experienced clinicians should be aware of false responses due to the natural discomfort of palpating these areas.

> **Box 15.3** Screening questions for suspected inflammatory back pain
>
> - Early morning stiffness, back and/or neck >30 min (mechanical back pain often lasts for a shorter time)
> - Pain improves with exercise? (mechanical is often worse)
> - Awake 2nd half of night with pain/stiffness?
> - Alternating buttock pain?
> - Age under 45 at onset? Frequently in twenties/thirties at onset (mechanical often has later onset)
> - Close relatives with inflammatory arthritis?
> - Better on gentle movement rather than rest? (mechanical often better at rest)
> - Stiffness after sitting? (mechanical often increased pain on sitting relieved by standing)
> - History of one or more the following might be present:
> - Iritis (painful inflamed eye)
> - Achilles tendonitis
> - Plantar fasciitis
> - Inflammatory bowel disease
> - Psoriasis

*Calin et al 1977, Rudwaleit et al 2005, Clemence 2010.*

- It is important to differentiate between mechanical and inflammatory causes of back pain and therefore screening questions need to be included in the assessment to identify undiagnosed inflammatory back pain (Box 15.3).

**Muscle function**

- In common with other conditions inflammatory arthritis is typically associated with reduced power and muscle control.
- This will be most evident to the patient as difficulty performing previously problem free functional activity.

**Fatigue**

- Fatigue reported within an inflammatory arthritis can be directly associated with the pathological process.
- It can also result from the 'deconditioning' effect of having a long-term heath problem (loss of aerobic fitness and muscle power).
- In addition reports of fatigue can be a physical description of psychological states such as depression.

## Red flags

In cases of acute back pain the following can indicate serious pathology:
- Past history of malignant cancer
- Progressive neurological symptoms
- Saddle anaesthesia, cauda equina syndrome
- Bladder or bowel dysfunction, especially alteration of sphincter control
- Fever and unexplained weight loss

- Structural deformity
- Systemically unwell, immunosuppression, drug abuse
- Constant progressive, non-mechanical pain
- Thoracic pain
- Violent trauma
- Age of onset less than 20 or more than 55 years.
- Prolonged use of corticosteroids (Moffett and McLean 2006).

### Specific red flags in rheumatoid arthritis
- Sepsis
- Drug toxicity
- Cervical spine instability
- Systemic rheumatoid vasculitis
- Unexplained weight loss and lymphadenopathy as a feature of other systemic disease, e.g. lymphoma or amyloid
- Exacerbations of respiratory or cardiac disease (Luqmani et al 2009).

## Other aspects of history taking

- It is standard practice within all areas of physiotherapy to record the patient's past medical history, current medication and social history.
- Social situation can affect and be affected by a rheumatological condition; given that most conditions are chronic, there can be long-term implications for maintaining social function.

## Symptom diaries

- Rheumatology patients who have diverse and variable symptoms or who are poor historians may be able to collect information about their symptoms by keeping a diary.
- This may delay completion of the initial assessment, but can provide much more coherent information about the symptoms being experienced by the patient.
- These have been used to gain a better understanding of pain presentation in oncology patients, respiratory tract illnesses and paediatric conditions (Schumacher et al 2002, Holmes et al 2001, Palermoa et al 2004).

## Drug history

- The drug history is of particular relevance in rheumatology because medication forms the basis of controlling the condition. Common areas for consideration follow.

## Phase of drug treatment

- Some drugs used in rheumatology have a time delay before therapeutic effects occur, e.g. methotrexate (one of the commonest used) can be up to 12 weeks.
- The patient's condition on later assessment might be different from initial contact if they have only just commenced medication at time of first contact.

## Corticosteroids

- These have the potential to rapidly suppress the inflammatory process and so are sometimes used as a short-term treatment to subdue a particularly aggressive acute inflammatory arthritis before the long-term treatment gains full effect.
- If a patient is assessed during the phase of maximum suppression from corticosteroids the clinician can sometimes gain a false impression about the presentation of the disease.

## Disruption of drug treatment

- Often this is due to problems with self-administered injections, home drug delivery, obtaining repeat prescriptions, misunderstanding about dose escalation, interruption of treatment and misunderstanding of previous advice.

## Drug side effects

- All drugs have side effects. It is outside the scope of practice for most physiotherapists to provide detailed advice about drug use for rheumatological conditions.
- If a problem is identified during assessment then it is important to liaise with the appropriate team member.
- Rheumatology departments will normally have specialist nurses who provide advice about medication.
- It is inadvisable for physiotherapists to use written sources such as a British National Formulary (BNF 2010) to resolve uncertainties.
- If in doubt seek advice.

## Objective assessment

- Objective examination in rheumatology shares much common ground with those conducted within general musculoskeletal practice and orthopaedics.
- The purpose of assessment is to identify the problems, understand their relevance to the patient, and formulate a plan for intervention.
- Currently there is no consensus about which is the most effective process for the assessment of patients who have known rheumatological conditions.
- The physiotherapist needs to make considered decisions about the objective information that needs to be gathered during the rheumatology assessment process.
- Physiotherapy assessment within rheumatology requires a sophisticated approach that is not compatible with asking the patient standard questions and performing set observations.
- Medical musculoskeletal examination has tended to follow the rough outline of 'look, feel, move' (Hassell and Cushnaghan 2010). However, conditions such as inflammatory arthritis or connective tissue disorders are diffuse diseases affecting other body systems alongside the musculoskeletal system and they can affect a number of areas of the body simultaneously.
- There is an inherent tension during the assessment between the need to get an overview of multiple functional problems and getting the specific information

about the issues affecting a single component within the musculoskeletal system.

- A skill that the rheumatology physiotherapist needs to develop is knowing what to include and what to leave out in the objective plan, a process that is constantly refined through the application of clinical reasoning and increasing experience.

## Observation

- The physiotherapist will need to decide how much of the patient they need to observe in order to inform clinical decision making. This decision will be made according to the purpose of the assessment.
- The patient needs to understand what the assessment will involve and consent to being assessed. Ideally the patient would be observed in standing from anterior, posterior and both lateral directions, in their underwear to visualise the limbs and skin surface (Box 15.4).
- An alternative to doing this is to observe different regions one at a time enabling the patient to remain covered in order to respect patient dignity or cultural needs.
- Patients with rheumatoid and psoriatic arthritis will often have hand joint involvement which can make dressing difficult, so this needs to be considered.

### The skin appearance
- Psoriasis, rashes, other skin lesions.

### Swelling, deformity, asymmetry, body shape or size
- It is also useful at this stage to note the overall appearance of the patient.
- When there are signs of poor personal care this can indicate potential problems with activities of daily living (ADL) due to joint dysfunction, especially hands or upper limbs.

## Assessment of movement (general)

- Time constraint or the acute nature of the patient's condition might mean that the physiotherapist will need to decide if they undertake a general screening with detailed assessment of specific areas.
- The patient can have inflammatory and degenerative changes in the same region or joint, and possibly changes due to trauma. Clinical reasoning process needs to consider these possibilities.
- The less experienced clinician is advised to consult more experienced colleagues, especially in the presence of a 'red flag'.
- Significant amounts of information can be gained from careful observation of active movement noting range, rhythm, ease of movement, painful arcs, 'trick movements' and inequalities of range between the different movements.
- Is it pain, weakness, joint stiffness or a mechanical block limiting movement and function? A judgement is needed about how much movement the patient can perform, based on the presentation of their condition.
- In the presence of an acute arthritis with widespread pain it might be inappropriate to do detailed tests of individual joint ranges. The assessment will require a functional orientation, e.g. general function, balance stability, walking ability and rising from lying and sitting. If a patient presents with acute

**Box 15.4** Observation (adapted from Arthritis Research UK 2011)

**In standing from head down**

General observation of body shape, size and appearance

Signs of general neglect

Skin, colour, condition

General symmetry

General speed and freedom of movement

Signs of surgery/trauma, scars

**Anterior and lateral views**

Cervical protrusion and lordosis (ankylosing spondylitis, cervical degeneration)

Cervical/shoulder asymmetry

'Dowager's hump'

Muscle spasm

Shoulder muscle bulk

Elbow flexion deformity

Lumbar lordosis

Hip flexion deformity

Quadriceps muscle bulk

Knee valgus/varus

Knee flexion deformity

Knee swelling

Ankle/forefoot positions/hindfoot/foot pronation/supination

Toe deformity/clawing/crossing

Toe dactylitis (inflammation of an entire digit)

**Posterior view**

Cervical position and symmetry

Shoulder muscle bulk and symmetry

Scapular position

Spinal alignment – scoliosis, iliac crest/posterior superior iliac spine symmetry

Elbow joint swelling

Gluteal muscle bulk

Posterior knee joint swelling

Calf muscle bulk

Ankle joint swelling

Ankle/hind foot position, over pronation, tendo-Achilles alignment

Weight distribution

**Wrist and hand**

These benefit from detailed observation and examination

Pattern and severity of joint swelling, finger dactylitis and skin changes

Deformities in established rheumatoid arthritis: ulnar deviation, swan neck and boutonniere deformities

Osteoarthritis: Heberden's nodes

arthritis then it is appropriate to liaise with the rheumatologist for information about the overall management plan.

- The time of day can affect the measurements obtained from those patients who have significant morning stiffness.

- Posture is a significant factor in inflammatory arthritis, e.g. ankylosing spondylitis (AS) and will influence the measurement of range of movement.

- A patient's perceptions, expectations and beliefs can have a very significant impact on what within physiotherapy is traditionally considered 'objective assessment'. Functional ability is a direct consequence of psychological processes and not just body biomechanics or physiology (Keefe and Somers 2010).

- Patients attend review assessments within rheumatology, therefore all measurements should be performed in a way which can be repeated at each review.

- Cardiac function may be tested by cardiologists and physiotherapists should be aware of the potential for cardiac and other systems to be involved in rheumatological conditions.

## Axial skeleton

### Active movements

- Cervical protraction and retraction can stress neck joints and should be used with caution if they need to be carried out.

- Curve reversal is an important point to note in the presence of spinal movements. With spinal stiffness in AS, a patient may display a good functional range of flexion whilst having a rigid lumbar spine, the movement being achieved entirely through motion at the hip joints.

- Cervical instability is a serious complication of rheumatoid arthritis and if suspected should be referred for a medical opinion. Physiotherapists should follow local policy and check red flags if planning to use manual techniques on the cervical spine in patients with inflammatory arthritis (Moffett and McLean 2006).

- In AS and the spondyloarthropathies the sternal, sternocostal, and costovertebral joints can all be involved, potentially affecting chest expansion. Measurement of chest expansion using a tape measure at xiphisternum level can be helpful to establish a baseline.

- Reduced rib joint flexibility causes reduction of respiratory efficiency and can reduce exercise tolerance. Selective testing of aerobic fitness can be useful in patients starting an aerobic exercise programme.

- In the majority of cases ankylosing spondylitis will begin in the sacroiliac joints and lumbar spine before the cervical spine. If AS is suspected in the lumbar spine then it is useful to undertake testing of the other vertebral regions because it might involve currently unaffected regions in the future.

- The Bath Ankylosing Spondylitis Metrology Index (BASMI) is a measurement tool (Table 15.2), which can provide an indication of the movement restrictions caused by AS and is used in the long-term review of the patient (Irons and Jeffries 2004).

- To determine the degree of limitation, add the 0, 1, 2 scores for each of the five measurements in Table 15.2 (the mean for cervical spine rotation counting as one score and similarly for tragus to wall and lumbar spine side flexion). This will provide a figure out of 10. This is the BASMI score. The higher the

**Table 15.2** Bath AS Metrology Index (BASMI), Jenkinson et al (1994)

|  | Mild 0 | Moderate 1 | Severe 2 |
|---|---|---|---|
| C. Spine Rotation (mean of R&L) | >70° | 20–70° | <20° |
| Tragus to wall (mean of R&L) | <15 cm | 15–30 cm | >30 cm |
| Lumbar side flexion (mean of R&L) | >10 cm | 5–10 cm | <5 cm |
| Lumbar flexion (modified Schobers) | >4 cm | 2–4 cm | <2 cm |
| Intermalleolar distance | >100 cm | 70–100 cm | <70 cm |

BASMI score the more severe the patient's limitation of movement due to their AS. An alternative scoring method can be found in Irons and Jeffries (2004).

- Most mechanical tests of the sacroiliac joints (SIJ) also put some stress on the hip or lumbar spine potentially making it hard to differentiate between these regions when more than one area has abnormalities. This is more likely to be the situation in older patients.

## Assessment of peripheral joints

- It can be challenging to select the tests which are most helpful in informing the assessment process, especially when degenerative changes can co-exist with inflammatory arthritis.

- The hands and feet are often among the first areas to be affected in inflammatory arthritis and in undiagnosed cases who present with bilateral joint signs and symptoms this can be among the first indications of a developing condition (NICE 2009).

- The pattern of joint involvement will differ between rheumatoid arthritis, psoriatic arthritis and osteoarthritis; however, older patients may have pre-existing degenerative changes. These need to be differentiated from the development of problems associated with an inflammatory arthritis. In patients where the presentation is unclear then it might be useful for the patient to have appropriate diagnostic tests (e.g. plain X-rays, MRI scan or an ultrasound scan).

- A variety of methods exist for detailed measurement of finger joint movement. When measuring individual joint ranges it is important to keep sight of the overall purpose of the assessment. A collection of joint ranges in degrees is meaningless unless it relates both to function and the physiotherapy intervention process.

- It is helpful to consider the range of basic grips performed by the hand and wrist. Assessment needs to be directed at the loss of ability to perform these grips along with other subtle functional hand actions such as pressing and pushing.

- There needs to be effective multidisciplinary team working, for example with OTs, if there is potential for their involvement. A clear understanding of how core physiotherapy skills can help in the team management of patients is essential.

- The lower limb requires testing in non-weight bearing and standing.

- Balance tests can be informative, observing stepping up and down on a step, rising from sitting and (with appropriate patients) standing on one leg can all reveal muscle weakness, poor coordination and balance.

- Single leg standing whist flexing and extending the weight-bearing leg can also give an indication of fine muscle control and balance in that limb. Remember rheumatoid arthritis can cause significant toe joint deformities, which can have Implications for balance.

- Biomechanical abnormalities can be helped by use of orthoses. Assessment for these is often provided by podiatry or orthotic services. The physiotherapist will need to liaise with the podiatrist or orthotist regarding the effectiveness of the orthotic.

## Palpation

- Palpation in rheumatology is used to detect the presence of synovitis in peripheral joints, i.e. warmth, pain and swelling. It is a skill which develops with practice and palpation for temperature change can be performed with the back of the hand for added sensitivity. A high degree of skill is needed to interpret palpation findings.

- A rheumatology body chart is a useful tool for recording findings when assessing the hands or feet (Figure 15.2, page 234).

- Palpation of specific joints forms part of the DAS 28 assessment indicating severity of the disease process (Wells et al 2009).

## Assessment format

### The use of assessment proformas

- This is almost universal within the physiotherapy profession in clinical practice. These are a compromise between gathering all relevant information and working within the limited time available during an appointment.

- Printed assessment paperwork needs to be regarded as a tool to support assessment, they should not dictate the clinical reasoning process.

- This is especially important in rheumatology, which often involves conditions which are chronic and affecting multiple areas of the body.

- It is not possible to use a template that will meet the requirements of every rheumatological presentation. However there are tools available that can assist the physiotherapist in selecting information from the objective assessment, e.g. 'GALS' locomotor screening (Doherty et al 1992).

### Example of upper limb rheumatology assessment formats

#### Standard format assessment headings

Name    Date of birth    Contact details

NHS/Hospital number

Social history:

Record symptoms (pain, paraesthesia, numbness) on standard body chart

24 hour pattern

General health, including red flags and drug history:

History of present condition:

Past medical history:

Upper limb objective assessment (lower limb form will be similar in format)

**Table 15.3** Recording assessment findings in the hand

| 5th digit | Active | Passive/accessory | Resisted |
|---|---|---|---|
| MCPJ | | | |
| PIPJ | | | |
| DIPJ | | | |
| **4th digit** | **Active** | **Passive/accessory** | **Resisted** |
| MCPJ | | | |
| PIPJ | | | |
| DIPJ | | | |
| **3rd digit** | **Active** | **Passive/accessory** | **Resisted** |
| MCPJ | | | |
| PIPJ | | | |
| DIPJ | | | |
| **2nd digit** | **Active** | **Passive/accessory** | **Resisted** |
| MCPJ | | | |
| PIPJ | | | |
| DIPJ | | | |
| **Thumb** | **Active** | **Passive/accessory** | **Resisted** |
| MCPJ | | | |
| IPJ | | | |

Observation:

Range of movement, recording range, quality of movement, limiting factors and symptoms during movement. A grid can be used to record the movements at each joint when carried out actively, passively and against resistance. Table 15.3 shows how this may be used for assessment of the hand. The same layout can be used for other areas such as the shoulder girdle or the hip.

Record additional notes, e.g. joint pattern, dactylitis, deformity.

Palpation: record findings on body chart.

Additional tests, e.g. neural assessment, neural dynamic testing

Special tests, e.g. joint integrity tests

Problem list

Treatment plan

### Enthesitis monitoring

Where enthesitis is suspected then it may be useful to use a specific tool such as the Mander Enthesis Index (MEI) (Mander et al 1987).

The following points are palpated and tenderness recorded:

- Iliac crest R and L
- Posterior superior iliac spine (psis) R and L
- Lumbar 5 spinous process
- Achilles insertion R and L
- 1st costochondral junction R and L
- 7th costochondral junction R and L
- Anterior superior iliac spine (asis) R and L

Tenderness on palpation of the points listed converts to a score with 0 (no points tender) to 13 (all points tender). Refer to Appendix 15.1 for an example of the enthesitis index.

The assessment findings should provide evidence-based information about the patient and their associated problems that will enable an appropriate treatment plan to be devised and implemented that is specific to the needs of each patient.

The references for this chapter can be found on www.expertconsult.com.

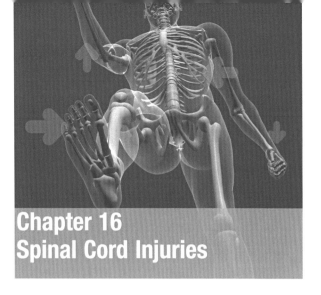

# Chapter 16
# Spinal Cord Injuries

## Acute spinal cord injuries

### Introduction

- A spinal cord injury (SCI) is a traumatic event for both the patient and their family and it provides a multifactorial challenge to health care staff.

- It is fortunately a relatively rare presentation, with approximately 800–1000 new cases per year and an estimated 40 000 people living with an SCI in the UK (Kennedy 1998, Nichols et al 2005, Harrison 2007).

- When compared to other neurological disorders, such as a cerebrovascular accident (CVA) – 150 000 cases/year in the UK (Carroll et al 2001), the chances of a student or Band 5 physiotherapist encountering a SCI patient outside of a specialist centre is slim.

- However, it is this unfamiliarity with the presentation that can be particularly daunting to a physiotherapist of any grade.

- Most new cases of SCI first present to a district general hospital via accident and emergency.

- The National Service Framework for Long Term Conditions (Department of Health 2005) suggests a minimum standard of up to 24 hours of diagnosis and transfer within the first 48 hours; admission to a specialist centre is likely to be delayed by concerns around medical stability and bed availability (Harrison 2007).

- Patients with an established injury are also likely to be admitted to their local hospital during periods of acute deterioration or other periods of illness.

- Some patients with dual diagnoses, e.g. SCI and a traumatic brain injury may never reach an SCI centre.

- This can also be the case with some patients that have non-traumatic spinal cord impairments.
- As such, the initial management will invariably be provided by a therapist with a generalised experience or no previous experience of working with patients that have incurred a spinal cord injury.
- In addition to the management required during the acute phase, immediately post injury, the patient will require longer-term rehabilitation.
- If the patient has been managed in a SCI centre during the acute phase they will require their care to be transferred to a hospital/service closer to their home, for management of their progression or maintenance of their presentation.
- This may include physiotherapy rehabilitation.
- With the muscle imbalance and overuse characteristics inherent in SCI, complaints of a musculoskeletal nature are also common (Bromley 2006).
- Thus, a physiotherapist is likely to be required to manage the care of a SCI patient in a number of different circumstances at some time in their career, regardless of their background being respiratory, neurological or musculoskeletal.
- It is therefore in a therapist's interest to develop a basic understanding of the presentation and needs of this patient population, and more importantly, a knowledge of where to seek and access assistance in the sometimes complex and challenging care that these patients need to receive.
- Therapists encountering patients with SCI for the first time can feel concerned that they do not have the appropriate clinical skills or knowledge to effectively manage this patient group.
- However it is important to stress at this point that a therapist should not consider that they are managing a patient in isolation.
- Specific advice should always be sought from SCI centres to ensure the patient is being managed in the best possible way and this will ensure that the therapist develops their experience, expertise and confidence in an appropriate way.
- Most SCI centres aim to provide acute outreach teams, either in person and/or via phone to advise, educate and support peer professionals.
- This service has been shown to improve referral times and reduce the incidence or severity of preventable complications prior to a patient's transfer (Harrison 2001, 2007).
- It cannot be emphasised enough that the information included in this book does not propose to replace the specific individualised advice that can be obtained from contacting specialists in the field of SCI management based in the 11 SCI centres in the UK (Appendix 16.1).
- However, the assessment of a patient with a spinal cord injury follows a fundamental construct, using the skills of assessment that are common to all physiotherapists, and the information obtained will provide the basis of the patient's planned management.
- The aim of this text is to demonstrate to a therapist new to the field that they already have many skills to assess and manage this presentation and with some background knowledge and slight adjustment to the delivery, a competent and effective delivery of care is achievable for an otherwise challenging presentation.

- A spinal cord injury is considered to be one of the most devastating conditions that can occur following a trauma.
- In seconds an individual is catapulted from a familiar life as an able-bodied person into a previously unknown situation and an environment of, in most cases, permanent disability.

## Mechanism and demographics

- The most common mechanism for a traumatic SCI is a sudden impact or deceleration whereby the forces are transmitted through the spinal column. Velocity is not related to the existence of injury, but will affect the extent of injury if one is to occur (Ravichandran 1990).
- Road traffic accidents, falls and injuries from participating in sport are the most common causes of SCI.
- Incidence of SCI in the British Isles is outlined in Table 16.1.
- Up to 50% of injuries from a motor vehicle collision will also present with multi-trauma, including multiple level spinal injury, limb fracture, abdominal, chest, facial or head injury or significant soft tissue trauma (Prasad et al 1999).
- Non-traumatic causes, e.g. neoplasm, infarct, infection, have been estimated at being 20% of the total prevalence (Harrison 2007).
- In a 5-year prospective study of the Irish National Spinal Unit between 1999 and 2003, Lenehan et al (2009) reported 73% of admissions were male, with an average age of 32 years.
- The majority were injuries to the cervical spine (51%), followed by lumbar (28%) and thoracic (21%).
- One third had a complete spinal injury on admission.
- Previously, the condition was predominantly seen in young men, but as the population ages and remains more active, there has been a discernable increase in the number of older people with SCI (Nichols et al 2005).
- Paralysis most frequently occurs in traumatic SCI when instability and damage to the spinal column leads to disruption of the spinal cord.
- 'Severance' or 'cutting' of the spinal cord rarely occurs outside of stabbing or gunshot injuries.
- More commonly, compression of the spinal cord resulting in ischaemic necrosis and swelling, leads to the formation of the impairment (Harrison 2007).

**Table 16.1** Causes of SCI in the United Kingdom & Ireland (O'Connor and Murray 2006)

| Cause of injury | Number of SCI centre admissions |
| --- | --- |
| Fall | 24 |
| Motor vehicle collision | 23 |
| Sport/recreation | 4 |
| Knocked over (e.g. falling object) | 1 |
| Other | 1 |

- It is thus difficult to predict the finality of the impairment, as the oedema and spinal shock can progress or resolve over time, with subsequent changes in neurological impairment (Ravichandran 1990).

## Initial management

- The spinal cord injured patient will present with a wide range of impairments that may include all of the body systems.
- Patients with an acute SCI will need specific management to stabilise the injury site and maintain the function of the vital systems of the body to prevent complications from occurring.
- Upon arrival to A&E, assessment of the person with suspected spinal cord injury will commence immediately by the medical team.
- Once vital signs and life-threatening concerns are dealt with, the doctor will assess the injury, looking for obvious signs of spinal injury, such as spinal deformity and pain on palpation, loss or altered power or sensation and bladder and bowel disturbance (Harrison 2007).
- There will typically follow a request for a spinal X-ray, computed tomography (CT) and magnetic resonance imaging (MRI) of the affected area to determine stability of the fracture and the extent of spinal cord damage.
- Clinically, this will be paralleled with a test to determine neurological level and the degree of completeness.
- The American Spinal Injury Association (ASIA) developed a classification which has been adopted internationally, to assess and monitor the spinal cord injury (Figure 16.1).
- The motor assessment assesses 10 key muscles bilaterally (5 in the upper limb, 5 in the lower limb) whilst the sensory assessment assesses each dermatome bilaterally using standardised anatomical landmarks for light touch and pin prick sensation.
- Combined together this information determines the neurological level of injury, the completeness of injury and the syndrome (if an incomplete injury is diagnosed).
- The 'neurological level' is defined as 'the lowest segment where motor and sensory function is normal on both sides' (ASIA 2001) or in other words, the last level of normal neurological function.
- This does not always correspond to the level of vertebral injury.
- The higher the injury level, the greater the number of bodily functions that will be adversely affected.
- Patients with incomplete spinal cord injuries may experience more pain and muscle imbalance than a patient with a complete lesion at the same level.
- The neurological level may change over time as the swelling or bleeding within the spinal cord develops.
- Should the level ascend, it will be an important indicator of the potential progression of a disease or the onset of a complication.
- This can occur in both acutely injured and established patients.
- Thus subjective reporting and clinical monitoring are vitally important in identifying the frequency with which the assessment monitoring should be carried out.

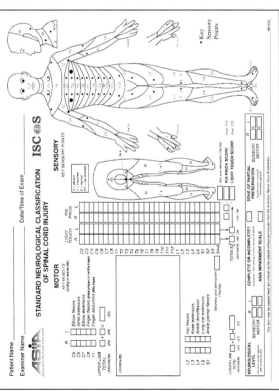

**Figure 16.1** Standards for Neurological Classification of SCI Worksheet (Dermatomes Chart). American Spinal Injury Association, 2011. *International Standards for Neurological Classification of Spinal Cord Injury, revised April, 2011.* American Spinal Injury Association, Chicago, IL. http://www.asia-spinalinjury.org/.

- Confusion often exists around the classification of complete versus incomplete injury.
- The ASIA Impairment Scale (AIS) provides a framework within which a categorisation can be provided.
- The scale is divided into five groups, A–E.
- Each of these is outlined on the reverse side of the standardised worksheet (Box 16.1).
- In the acute phase the exact extent of the completeness of the lesion may not be clearly defined due to the presence of swelling surrounding the spinal cord.

## Complete lesion
- AIS grade A
- This classification is given in the absence of S4/5 sensory and motor preservation.
- It is possible, nonetheless, to include 'zones of partial preservation'.

## Zones of partial preservation
- Some people present with unilateral or bilateral function below the level of the injury site, without preservation of S4/5 function.
- These segments are described as 'zones of partial preservation' and can be either sensory and/or motor in function.

---

**Box 16.1** Categorisation of SCI

A = Complete:

No motor or sensory function is preserved in the sacral segments S4 to S5

B = Incomplete:

Sensory but not motor function is preserved below the neurological level and includes the sacral segments S4 to S5

C = Incomplete:

Motor function is preserved below the neurological level and more than half of the key muscles below the neurological level have a muscle grade less than 3

D = Incomplete:

Motor function is preserved below the neurological level and at least half the key muscles below the neurological level have a muscle grade of 3 or more

E = Normal:

Motor and sensory function are normal

**Clinical syndromes**

Central cord

Brown Sequard

Anterior cord

Conus medullaris

Cauda equina

---

*American Spinal Injury Association: International Standards for Neurological Classification of Spinal Cord Injury, revised 2011: Atlanta, GA. Reprinted 2011.*

## Incomplete lesion

- This includes AIS grades B–D.
- Sacral function at S4/5 must be preserved.
- The classification ASIA E is used for those who have normal motor function within the key muscles and normal sensory function.
- The motor and sensory scoring, however, may not be sensitive enough to identify the presence of spasticity or pain, subtle weakness, core instability or certain forms of dysaesthesia that could be a result of a spinal cord injury.
- Therefore those who are categorised AIS E may still require rehabilitation to address these issues.

## Spinal shock

- Following a SCI, there will be a sudden and transient suppression of both somatomotor reflexes and autonomic function below the injury.
- This 'spinal areflexia' will result in flaccid paralysis of trunk and limbs and loss of vasomotor function with resultant hypotension.
- Urinary retention and constipation ensue due to bladder and bowel stasis (known as 'paralytic ileus') and male patients may experience sustained priapism (Nichols et al 2005).
- Perhaps the most worrying component for the physiotherapist is the loss of sympathetic outflow to the heart in injuries above T3, resulting in bradycardia or sinus arrest during turns, and suctioning. However, this is preventable.
- The period of spinal shock can last up to 6 weeks, but can be delayed by post injury complications (Benevento and Sipski 2002).
- Resolution of certain reflexes occurs at different rates, with Babinski's sign returning within the first day and bladder tone requiring up to 3 months (Ditunno et al 2004).

## Autonomic dysreflexia

- This is a potentially fatal consequence of an injury above T6.
- It is the body's exaggerated reaction to a noxious stimulus below the neurological level, resulting in a rapid and extreme increase in blood pressure, which, if untreated, could cause cerebral haemorrhage.
- It manifests with a pounding headache, sweating and blotching of the skin above the lesion, pallor below the lesion, and bradycardia (Nichols et al 2005).
- The stimulus is usually a blocked catheter, constipation, sharp object, labour or passive movements.
- Treatment includes removing the stimulus, sitting the patient upright and using antihypertensive medication, e.g. nitrolingual spray.

## Heterotrophic ossification

- Abnormal calcification at areas of small muscle tears is a suggested aetiology of this presentation, whereby bone is deposited around joints, especially the hip and knees.
- However the pathophysiology is still a matter for conjecture.
- The first signs are a 'spongy' end feel, with mild oedema and erythema.

- X-rays are normal for the first 2–3 weeks, then show 'cloudy patches' in affected areas (Bromley 2006).
- Ultrasonography is the preferred diagnostic tool in early stages and epidronate is the medication of choice.
- Passive movements are discontinued initially for approximately 1 week. Frequency, repetition and force of passive movements are progressed cautiously over the ensuing 4–8 weeks (Bromley 2006).
- Surgery is only considered in cases of hindered function and/or sitting posture, however recurrence of ossification at the surgical site is common.

## Syringomyelia

- This is a fluid-filled cavity within the spinal parenchyma which forms due to impaired CSF flow, predominantly due to mechanical encroachment, redirecting flow into the cord.
- It is evidenced by localised pain, tonal alteration and ascension of neurological level in established patients (Bromley 2006).
- Diagnosis is by MRI and management either involves monitoring or insertion of a surgical shunt.
- Effectiveness of either approach is highly variable and remains a topic for discussion.

### Other complications

- The multisystem impairment involved in a spinal injury predisposes a patient to a wide variety of other complications.
- The most common include:
- Recurrent urinary tract infections
- Abdominal distension
- Contracture
- Postural deformation
- Spasticity
- Pain
- Pressure sores
- Cardiovascular compromise
- Osteoporosis (Bromley 2006).
- The physiotherapist must be mindful of the potential or presence of these as it will alter the assessment and future preventative or curative management offered.

## Planning and implementing the assessment of SCI

- The physiotherapist must draw on their knowledge of anatomy, physiology and the core areas of their training in cardiorespiratory, musculoskeletal and neurological assessment approaches when approaching the assessment of a patient with a SCI.
- Therapists new to the field may feel overwhelmed by the number of impairments affecting a patient and not know where to start.

- It is therefore important to use a problem list approach to organise the process of applying clinical reasoning and problem solving.
- This will ensure that no important components of the assessment or issues are accidentally missed.
- It is the practice at the National Spinal Injuries Centre (NSIC) at Stoke Mandeville to use a set format to guide the assessment and treatment planning, these will include the following:
- Respiratory (always the first priority)
- Range of motion/muscle length
- Sensation
- Muscle power
- Tone
- Pain
- Skin
- Residual function and abnormal patterns of movement
- Psychology and cognition
- Functional assessment
- Cardiovascular fitness.
- The reader should recognise that they already have many skills from their core training and previous clinical experiences that they can utilise to address the areas identified in the list.
- These skills remain valid and with some modification can be used in the assessment of this patient population with its specific needs.
- A clinician with little experience of working with SCI patients will soon find that they are able to undertake a comprehensive and effective assessment and formulate a treatment plan for a patient with a complex presentation.
- The headings from the list will be covered later in the chapter to illustrate how the therapist may assess the specific needs of the SCI patient and how this information may be used to ensure that the treatment plan is 'spinal specific'.

## Acute stage (bedrest) assessment

- Physiotherapy will commence as soon after the patient's admission as possible in conjunction with the plan for the chosen form of medical management.
- Either surgical or conservative management of a spinal fracture may be considered.
- This will determine the length of bedrest that is required following injury and can influence the sequence of rehabilitation, but should not dramatically change the outcome of rehabilitation.
- Whilst the spine is still considered 'unstable' a patient will be nursed in a supported bed (Figure 16.2a, b).
- A turning bed is the treatment of choice to decrease carer load whilst ensuring spinal alignment and respiratory and skin integrity.
- The spine will be managed with either skull traction (Figure 16.3a), head blocks (Figure 16.3b), cervical collar or pillows for postural reduction of spinal misalignment.
- Regular assessment of the patient forms an integral part of the treatment by the physiotherapist.

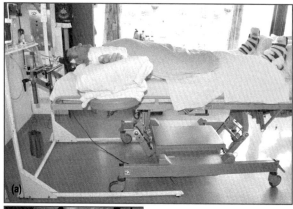

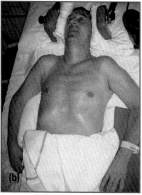

**Figure 16.2** (a) Patient in support position in bed. (b) Supported position in bed.

- Frequent review, re-evaluation and setting of goals is necessary to ensure treatment is effective and that the patient is involved in their rehabilitation as far as is practically possible.
- This philosophy should be followed throughout every patient's rehabilitation.
- The physiotherapist needs to carry out their own assessment of the patient as soon as possible with the evaluation of respiratory function being the first priority.
- Muscle power should be assessed and recorded regularly, especially if the neurological level is changing.
- Any change must be reported to the medical staff immediately.
- Prior to approaching the patient, the therapist must first ascertain the mechanism and level of injury, as well as the planned management.
- It is important to be familiar with the presence of any associated injuries, especially if they will alter the assessment, e.g. a limb or rib fracture.
- The patient's doctor should be questioned about the anticoagulation status prior to any limb movements, to minimise the risk of dislodging a thrombus.

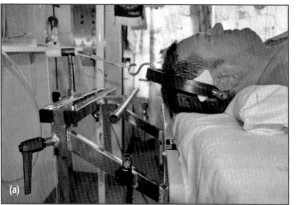

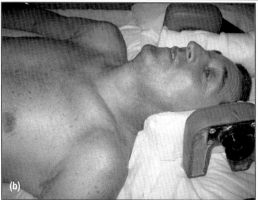

**Figure 16.3** (a) Skull traction. (b) Headblock immobilisation.

- With each precaution and contraindication considered, the therapist is ready to proceed with a structured assessment.

## Respiratory function

- The amount of chest physiotherapy required in the acute stage will depend on several factors:
- Level of spinal lesion
- Degree of completeness/incompleteness of spinal lesion
- Any associated injuries, e.g. haemothorax, fractured ribs
- Post injury complications, e.g. pneumonia, aspiration
- Previous respiratory pathology, e.g. chronic obstructive airways disease, heavy smoking history.

- The associated mechanical inefficiency of breathing often results with a potential for fatigue.
- This may lead to the patient requiring either non-invasive or invasive mechanical ventilation.
- This risk is highest during the period of spinal shock (due to chest wall flaccidity), or post fixation (due to pain and general anaesthesia).
- It is common to observe a patient compensating well over the first few days post injury, followed by a rapid deterioration as fatigue ensues.
- Cohen et al (1982) demonstrated that an increase in respiratory rate was the first sign of respiratory fatigue, prior to seeing changes in vital capacity.

## Assessment

- This will include general observation, auscultation, consulting chest X-rays, monitoring blood gas results and regular monitoring of vital capacity, which is imperative when paralysis of respiratory musculature is present. It should be noted that auscultation used in isolation can be misleading, as a low-volume inspiration may not allow the listener to hear all potential impairments.
- The inability of patients without innervation of abdominal muscles (typically T6 and above) to cough effectively will necessitate the use of forced expiratory techniques, such as assisted coughing. A therapist should thus routinely assess an independent cough, followed by noting the effectiveness of an assisted cough. The quality of sputum produced, if any, should also be noted.
- Palpation and identification of preserved respiratory muscle innervation is very important in the ultrahigh lesion as this will allow a therapist to predict a patient's potential to wean off ventilation or 'rescue breathe'.
- Any accompanying contraindications must be considered and appropriate modifications to assessment and eventual treatment must be made.

## Range of motion

- Following spinal cord injury, disruption of descending control and input to spinal motor neurones leads to muscle paralysis and weakness.
- Immobility follows and where there is some preserved muscular innervation around a joint, muscle imbalance occurs.
- Secondary structural changes occur as a result of weakness, immobilisation (which can be imposed for management of the unstable spine), pain and disuse. This can include muscular, capsular and ligamentous shortening and changes in muscle stiffness.
- These structural changes subsequently impose further restrictions to movement, described by Gracies as the 'paresis–disuse–paresis' cycle (Gracies 2005).
- An assessment of the patient's baseline joint range of motion must be carried out at this stage and should be monitored on a regular basis, especially when changes are suspected.
- Even the smallest loss of range can significantly limit functional outcome, e.g. restricted elbow extension for a complete C6 tetraplegic will restrict their ability to transfer independently or shortened hip flexor muscles will prevent a paraplegic from ambulating with calipers, whilst shortened hip adductor and rotator muscles will limit the level of independence a person

with spinal cord injury may achieve during activities of daily living such as lower body dressing.

- It must be remembered that restrictions to movement may be in place for the management of the unstable spine and therefore it may not be possible to fully assess the range of motion at every joint. Hip flexion is typically limited to 30° in unstable fractures at T10 and below, however full knee flexion range can be assessed by combining it with lateral rotation of the hip (i.e. the 'half tailor position') (Bromley 2006). Full shoulder range is essential for functional outcome, thus assessment should only be limited if it increases pain at the fracture site in an unstable cervical injury.

## Sensation

- The ASIA neurological assessment completed on admission including light touch and pin prick sensation of each dermatome provides useful information for the therapist also and can be a prognostic indicator, e.g. preservation of pin prick has been linked to a likelihood of motor recovery (Srivastava 2005).
- Proprioception is tested and tactile discrimination, temperature and stereognosis can also be useful.

## Muscle power

- The physiotherapist requires more in-depth information about muscle power than the 10 key muscles assessed by the medical team.
- Therefore a full muscle power assessment should be completed, in order to develop a treatment plan appropriate to the needs of the patient.
- The universal Oxford scale should be used and standardised as much as possible by the following means:
  - The patient must be able to complete the movement a minimum of three times through the full available range of motion in order to achieve the grade
  - If this is not possible, the lower grade should be given
  - Each muscle should be tested from the neutral position
  - Visualisation of the limb by the patient must be encouraged, if possible, in areas where proprioception is impaired
  - Assessment should commence with the grade 3 position and then be adjusted as necessary
  - + or − should not be used as this is highly subjective
  - Use of compensations (e.g. 'trick elbow extension') is common, but a therapist's handling can limit these, allowing a true picture of underlying muscle contraction.
- Whilst a patient is on bedrest and subject to movement restrictions, it may not always be possible to fully assess muscle power, i.e. assessment in a position against gravity may not be possible. In this instance common sense is required, but if there is any uncertainty, the lower grade is awarded.
- The initial assessment may need to be modified due to the fracture or associated injuries.
- The stability at the fracture site may be put in jeopardy should excessive force be used to complete the muscle power testing, therefore great care must be taken to avoid this.

- A number of other factors may influence the ability to test and the outcome therefore must be considered:
- Movement limitations, presence of brace or collar
- Pre-existing conditions
- Pain
- Fatigue
- Hypertonia
- Medication
- Psychological factors.

## Tone assessment

- Hypertonia is a common consequence of spinal cord injury, especially those with incomplete SCI, grades B and C (Heckman 1994).
- During spinal shock, the limbs are flaccid.
- As reflex activity returns, the emergence of altered tone may become evident.
- This may occur earlier and more significantly in patients with an incomplete lesion. Spasticity tends to gradually increase over the first year post injury before it plateaus.
- The neurophysiology of hypertonia is complex and encompasses both neural and non-neural (atrophy, change in number of sarcomeres, changes in muscle fibre type, intrinsic stiffness, muscle receptors) components.
- The management of the neural components is primarily pharmacological, whilst the management of the non-neural factors is through therapy and positioning and it is these factors that are considered to be the major cause of disability.
- Spasticity can be elicited by many stimuli, with touch and stretch being the most common, but infection, illness, injury or an overdistended bladder or bowel can also give rise to spasticity.
- It is therefore important to try to establish the potential cause and contribution of neural and non-neural factors in eliciting spasticity to aid with the control and management of this problem.
- There are a multitude of measures that can be used to assess and document tone, the most widely used are the Modified Ashworth score and the Tardieu scale.
- The presence of hypertonia can impact significantly on function and information regarding functional restrictions imposed by hypertonia can provide a very useful assessment and monitoring tool.
- Careful handling of the affected parts of the body is required and can provide a wealth of information on its own.

## Pain

- Pain is a common complication following spinal cord injury (SCI), which can limit participation in rehabilitation, ability to perform functional activities and can impact on the patient's quality of life.
- The location, intensity, time since onset of spinal cord injury, duration, cause and aggravating factors are highly variable.

- Kennedy et al (1998) found that 'pain at 6 weeks post injury is the strongest predictor of pain at one year post discharge.'
- There are a number of different types of pain commonly encountered following SCI.
- Siddall and Middleton (2006) classified pain into two distinct categories:
- Neuropathic pain, which is initiated or caused by a primary injury or dysfunction of the nervous system
- Nociceptive pain, which can be musculoskeletal or visceral in origin.
- Acute musculoskeletal pain arises from damage to anatomical structures and is often related to activity, position or muscle imbalance.
- Chronic musculoskeletal pain may occur with overuse or abnormal use of structures such as the arm or hand.
- Successful management is dependent upon early intervention and relies upon an accurate assessment and close monitoring of the pain. A body chart, like those used in musculoskeletal departments, is a simple and typical way to document this assessment.

## Skin condition

- SCI patients are particularly vulnerable to deterioration of the skin due to their altered circulation, sensation, muscle tone and functional capacity.
- A therapist involved in seating provision or the initial teaching of transfers must monitor the effect these have on the skin to avoid breakdown or further impairment.
- Documenting site, size and grading of a sore is typically sufficient for a therapist.

## Residual function and abnormal patterns of movement

- The levels of residual function will need to be determined during the acute stage, which will assist the physiotherapist to plan the treatment to encompass the remaining intact muscle groups.
- It is also important to note how abnormal patterns of movement interfere with the residual functional abilities of the patient and how easily these patterns can be modified.
- The early involvement of the patient in exercise and education can help prepare them as an individual to participate in the future goals of their rehabilitation.

## Psychology and cognition

- The psychological impact of spinal cord injury can never be overestimated.
- The physiotherapist may become aware of changes in a patient's mood and it is important that this is brought to the attention of the team members with specific skills in psychological assessment and management.
- The ability of the patient to engage with instructions will also have a bearing on their ability to achieve the high levels of independent function required during their rehabilitation. Impaired cognition may have been a causative factor in the spinal injury, or may have developed as a result (e.g. head injury or medication).

## Assessment for early rehabilitation

- The patient is allowed to mobilise once the spinal fracture is stable or they are deemed medically stable.
- Support for a fracture may be required in the form of a collar or spinal corset, which will be advised by the medical team.
- Appropriate cushioning and wheelchair mobility will need to be provided.
- Following mobilisation re-examination needs to be carried out.
- Due to the removal of many of the limitations that are imposed during the bed rest phase, e.g. positioning and factors to protect the unstable spine, there may be changes in the assessment findings.
- There may be changes in range of movement, muscle power, tone and pain. Improvements in strength could be due to neurological development or improved pain/cooperation, whilst an apparent deterioration could be due to the tester's ability to grade each muscle in the correct position.
- There may also be an organic cause and the reason for any deterioration must be documented and communicated to the appropriate medical staff.
- The patient's core control can be assessed once they are sitting up out of bed.
- It is at this stage that the rehabilitation potential is often defined.
- Physiotherapy assessment will re-evaluate the tests carried out in the initial assessment, identifying any complications and also the potential for functional development. Typically, this is performed once the patient can sit for longer than 4 hours, to counteract any effect fatigue may contribute.

## Functional assessment

- A functional assessment must take place for those commencing rehabilitation, those undertaking advanced rehabilitation or for those who require a further period of rehabilitation following a complication, illness or change in neurological status.
- The findings can be used to formulate a treatment plan, set appropriate goals, evaluate the efficacy of intervention and to engage and motivate the patient and family in the rehabilitation process.
- Functional assessment should form an integral part of rehabilitation and be completed on a regular basis.
- An understanding of the functional potential for each spinal level and an awareness of the potential complications and limitations is required to tailor the functional assessment and formulate the treatment plan. This is outlined in Appendix 16.3. The current ability and predicted level of independence of each of the following areas must be assessed and evaluated, documented and used to develop a treatment plan. Any limiting or interfering factors need to be assessed and minimised as part of the treatment plan.

## Wheelchair mobility

- The patient must be assessed for their ability to negotiate slopes, kerbs and uneven surfaces in addition to pushing on level surfaces including carpets etc.

- The technique of propulsion is also important to assess to identify poor technique which may lead to shoulder and upper limb pain and injury in the future.

## Gait assessment

- The assessment of gait following spinal cord injury falls into 2 categories:
- Patients with lower limb paralysis requiring orthoses to ambulate
- Patients with an incomplete spinal cord injury resulting in varying degrees of partial paralysis of the lower limb, who may also require orthoses.
- It is essential to be able to analyse the gait pattern of both the categories above to prevent injury, ensure efficiency and maximise function.
- It is also important to appreciate the role that extensor hypertonus may play in enabling some patients to walk. Whilst it is important to facilitate a normal pattern of extensor activity, over inhibition of the hypertonus may prevent the patient from mobilising.
- Knowledge of a normal gait pattern is crucial to be able to identify an abnormal gait pattern and numerous texts are available to provide this information. For further information regarding gait assessment for those with lower limb paralysis please consult (Bromley, 2006; Harvey, 2008).

## Potential for involvement in sport and work

During the rehabilitation process the patient may identify a wish to participate in sports and also the possibility of returning to work.

## Balance

- Balance forms an integral part of most activities, either in or out of the wheelchair.
- Balance in long sitting is required for many activities on the bed such as dressing, moving around the bed and moving from lying to sitting.
- Long sitting can also be used as a means of transferring, whilst balance in short sitting is often used for activities in the wheelchair, transfers, toileting, showering and dressing.
- The ability to maintain balance in long and short sitting as well as during a functional task must be assessed.
- The ability to maintain balance in the wheelchair during wheeled movement is a key component of the activities of daily living.
- Assessment must consider potential for independent propulsion, wheelchair management and the most appropriate seating system.

## Matwork

- Rolling, lying to and from sitting and moving around the bed form many of the components required for functional activities, e.g. dressing, turning in bed, getting in and out of bed and positioning pillows.
- The ability to complete the tasks and each individual component forms part of the overall assessment and can be used to indicate the level of care that may be required on discharge.

## Pressure relief and skin management

- A patient must become independent in being able to check their skin to ensure that it remains healthy and free from damage that could lead to infection and a return to bedrest.

- A patient's ability to visualise pressure areas with a mirror should be assessed as well as their independence in relieving pressure whilst in the wheelchair. Where physical independence is not achievable, verbal independence should be assessed instead.

## Transfers

- Prior to assessing any transfer a risk assessment must be undertaken to ensure safety for both the patient and the physiotherapist.

- Position of the wheelchair and sliding board (if used), alignment of the castors, starting and finishing position, hand position and body position during the transfer will have a significant effect on the ability to complete level transfers such as wheelchair to bed, split-level transfers and advanced transfers such as bath, toilet, car, floor and sofa.

- Therefore not only must the level of independence be assessed, but each of the component parts to ensure safe completion of the task and to prolong the ability to complete the task and avoid injury.

## Cardiovascular fitness

- Poor cardiovascular fitness is a leading cause of death post SCI. Cardus et al (1992) reported it was responsible for 50% of deaths.

- It also prevents patients performing many of the motor tasks that are required of them on a day-to-day basis (Harvey 2008).

- Stewart et al (2000) investigated a number of different objective assessments of fitness in the spinal population. Power output and $VO_2$ at maximal workload, and ratings of perceived exertion at a standard workload demonstrated stability and sensitivity to therapeutic change, much more so than HR or other ventilatory measures such as vital capacity. It should thus be considered that using the Borg Scale of Perceived Exertion is likely to be the most accurate and easy-to-use measure in the clinical context.

The references for this chapter can be found on www.expertconsult.com.

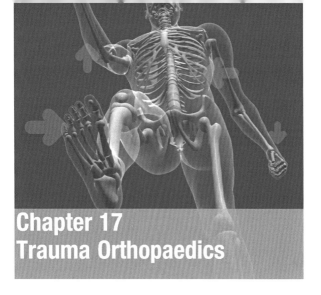

# Chapter 17
# Trauma Orthopaedics

## In-patients

- Trauma orthopaedics covers a multitude of injuries that are admitted to hospital in varying ways.

- It can range from those patients who walk in via Accident and Emergency (A&E) or fracture clinic with minor injuries, to those that are brought in by ambulance with life-threatening multi-trauma injuries.

- No matter how they arrive their assessment starts as soon as they enter the doors of the hospital.

- A doctor will always admit the patient and collect a lot of useful information that you as a physiotherapist will need to know prior to assessing a patient.

- This will not be an exhaustive list, therefore it is essential that a thorough subjective assessment is carried out.

- Due to the high-energy nature of many of the injuries encountered on a trauma orthopaedic ward, it is likely that your patient will present with multiple injuries.

- A common mistake in assessment of trauma orthopaedic patients is to concentrate on their obvious injury.

- Because fractures are extremely painful, it is quite common for a soft tissue injury to be missed initially and only to be discovered at a later date, e.g. a patient may present with a tibial shaft fracture; however, the less obvious rupture of the posterior cruciate ligament may be missed.

- It is often a physiotherapist that discovers these secondary injuries.

- Because of this it is essential to complete a thorough subjective and objective examination of all limbs, in addition to the patient's 'obvious' injury.

- Many patients who are admitted to a trauma ward will have associated wound and plastics issues from open fractures or fasciotomies.

- This is covered in Chapter 4 in this volume and in Volume 2.

- Unlike elective orthopaedics or sports physiotherapy, you will see many patients that have been admitted to hospital following severe accidents.
- The patient may have difficulty talking about their accident in circumstances where they have been involved in a fatal collision possibly involving other family members or where they feel at fault for their accident.
- This will affect patients in different ways, so they must be approached in a caring manner respecting their right to decide when they are ready to start physiotherapy.
- In this chapter the assessment approach covers the period from when the patient is admitted to hospital through to their discharge and subsequent referral to outpatient physiotherapy.

## Subjective assessment

- Like any acute ward, there are many different places to gather information about a patient, e.g. medical notes; doctor's admission sheet; talking to the patient's nurse and other members of the multidisciplinary team and X-rays.
- It is essential to realise that the subjective examination is an ongoing process and it is not always possible to collect all of the information from a patient on the first day. There are a wide variety of reasons that may prevent you from completing your assessment, such as drowsiness from anaesthesia, pain or confusion due to a head injury or dementia.
- In these cases, if possible, look to find out more information from their relatives or friends.
- In trauma orthopaedics, the type of information that is required may be similar to that required in other clinical settings that enable a clinical picture to be established. Examples of the questions specific to the trauma setting are outlined in Table 17.1.
- Once the subjective assessment has been completed, this should enable the objective assessment to be planned and the formulation of ideas relating to the patient's treatment goals and their discharge plan.

## Objective assessment

- It may not be possible to carry out a full objective assessment on the first day.
- This can be an ongoing process that will continue through to discharge.
- The objective assessment will generally follow a standard manual therapy format along the lines of a musculoskeletal textbook (Petty 2006).
- As patients will have different injuries and post operative instructions, it is essential to make the assessment specific to individual circumstances.
- If a patient requires an operation, then both preoperative and postoperative assessment will need to be completed.
- The areas commonly requiring assessment are as follows.

### Pain

- Pain is a big issue following a traumatic injury and subsequent surgery.
- The amount of pain can be evaluated using various tools, e.g. Visual Analogue Scale (VAS).

**Table 17.1** A range of trauma-specific questions used during subjective assessment

| Information | Questions |
|---|---|
| Mechanism of injury | Was it a high-energy injury such as a car crash or a low energy injury such as a simple fall? |
| Area and type of fracture | Which part of the body is affected?<br>Was it an open or closed fracture?<br>Was it a simple transverse or a multifragmented spiral fracture? |
| Treatment method | Is it non-operative or operative?<br>Are there any casts or braces needed? |
| Past medical history | Does your patient have any condition that will impact on their rehabilitation?<br>See trauma outpatient section for good examples of this |
| Previous mobility | Were they:<br>independent with no aids?<br>using a frame?<br>having recurrent falls?<br>Can they do stairs? |
| Previous ROM/ strength | Were they normally fit and healthy or do they have contractures or weakness? |
| Neurovascular status | Have they had previous vascular issues due to diabetes or do they normally have a foot drop? |
| Social history | What job do they need to get back to?<br>Do they:<br>play sport?<br>live alone?<br>have carers?<br>have children?<br>live in a house with stairs? |
| Drug history | What medications are they normally on?<br>Are they a drug user? |

- It is essential to assess a patient when they are covered by pain relief, to ensure information gained is as reliable as possible.

- If the patient experiences too much pain to continue then it is possible to request additional pain relief from the nursing staff, or alternatively return to see the patient later when their pain is under control.

## Imaging

- A major part of assessment will be reviewing and understanding any imaging the patient may have had.

- The most common images are X-rays, computerised tomography scans (CT scans), ultrasound scans and magnetic resonance imaging (MRI); Table 17.2, outlines where these may be used.

**Table 17.2** Imaging and examples of use

| Imaging type | Examples of use |
|---|---|
| X-rays | Initial imaging for suspected fracture/s |
| CT | Provides a better understanding of the extent of a fracture and potential management, e.g. a multi-fragmented tibial plateau fracture |
| Ultrasound | Tendon ruptures, e.g. quadriceps tendon<br>To determine soft tissue injury in a joint, e.g. ACL rupture |
| MRI | Assess neurological injury, e.g. sub-dural haematoma or spinal cord injury<br>To visualise a fracture if not visible on X-ray, e.g. undisplaced hip fracture |

- A physiotherapist will be expected to be able to examine an X-ray and determine whether it is normal or not.
- Although it is useful to be able to interpret CT and MRI scans, it is not expected that physiotherapists will be able to read these.
- A radiologist will review and report on all imaging and this will be a useful adjunct to the assessment.

## Observation

- Assessment begins as soon as the patient is seen.
- It is good practice to stand at the end of a patient's bed and observe the following:
- Position they are in
- Any drains or lines that are attached to them
- Their limb position
- Any swelling? If so where
- What casts, splints or braces they have
- Any traction in place
- Red swollen areas, question whether this is due to infection, especially if stitches are in situ.
- If the wound is covered in a dressing it is essential to notify the patient's nurse so that the dressing can be taken down and the cause established.

## Palpation

- It is good practice to palpate the patient's affected and unaffected limb.
- Assess for any differences in size due to swelling or muscle wastage, any hot and inflamed areas and any tender areas.
- Good palpation can often lead to diagnosis of complications that can arise due to the patient's injuries, e.g. compartment syndrome or deep vein thrombosis.

## Chest assessment

- Most patients that are admitted to a trauma ward will need a routine chest assessment for a variety of reasons.
- Previous respiratory history
- Prolonged bed rest due to their injury
- Administration of a general anaesthetic
- Admission with chest trauma, e.g. rib fractures, pneumothorax, haemothorax or lung contusions.
- If a patient is due an operation, then it is prudent to assess their chest pre- and postoperatively.

## Neurovascular status

- Due to the high-energy nature of traumatic injuries, pre- and postoperative assessment of a patient's neurovascular status is often required.
- Neurological damage can be due to a head injury, a spinal cord injury or a peripheral nerve injury.
- The physiotherapist should routinely consider if there are any abnormal sensation, altered pulses, loss of bladder or bowel control or power loss.
- Findings (positive or negative) must be recorded, to assist with identification of the cause of any neuropathy.
- This is especially important for patients with spinal injuries.
- It will help to monitor changes in a patient's neurological symptoms as a result of surgery.
- Follow the standard neurological assessment as described in a textbook to assess a patient's neurological status (Petty 2006).
- Any neurological symptoms should be recorded on a body chart and muscle chart. These can be filled out preoperatively, postoperatively and at regular intervals until symptoms have normalised or plateaued.
- In the case of spinal injuries, an American Spinal Injury Association (ASIA) score should be completed (http://www.asia-spinalinjury.org/).
- Swelling is a common outcome of traumatic injuries and operative procedures, entailing assessment of a patient's vascular system.
- This can be as simple as checking for abnormal skin colour, skin temperature and capillary refill.
- In the acute phase, any abnormal neurovascular status must be reported to a doctor immediately, in case it is due to a limb-threatening condition, e.g. compartment syndrome.

## Range of motion (ROM)

- Before assessing ROM of any joint, check for any restrictions imposed by the surgeon.
- Example of instructions could be:
- No movement at all, e.g. wearing a non-removable cast for 6 weeks or a backslab for a week to allow wounds to settle
- Restricted range of motion in a brace e.g. 0–30° for 2 weeks following a patella tendon repair
- Full active ROM, but no passive ROM.

- Measure range using a goniometer and avoid 'eye balling' ROM.
- If the patient is not allowed to move their affected limb, it is still essential to assess and document the ROM of their unaffected joints.
- Most patients will have reduced ROM and it is necessary to document any reasons for this, e.g. swelling, wound position, dressings or pain.
- If a wound is found to be oozing, then immediately inform the patient's nurse.

## Muscle power

- Assessing muscle power of the affected limb can be difficult in the acute trauma setting as there are many factors that will affect strength, such as pain, swelling, dressings and wounds.
- Look out for any external agents that can reduce muscle power such as epidurals or nerve blocks used during surgery.
- With this in mind, test each muscle methodically and document any muscles testing weak using the Oxford scale (Kendall and McCreary 2005).
- Patients can become weaker due to prolonged bed rest, therefore it is essential to assess the muscle power in all of the unaffected limbs as well.

## Function

- Assessing a patient's functional mobility is a major component of the assessment, which enables the therapist to inform nursing staff how to transfer them.
- The information will also inform the patient's treatment and discharge plan.
- Be aware of any restrictions that the patient may have from their injuries and subsequent operations or from previous medical conditions, e.g. a 60-year-old man with a fractured patella may be restricted by a knee brace to prevent knee flexion and a previous stroke that has left him with a hemiparesis.
- Functional tasks include the following:
- Rolling
- Bed transfers
- Sitting balance
- Sit to stand
- Standing balance
- Transfers
- Mobility
- Stairs.
- Whilst assessing these different functions consider the following:
- Amount of assistance needed, both in numbers and physical demand, e.g. moderate assistance of two people
- Side of the bed they are transferring from and to
- Any equipment that may be required such as bed levers, frames or wheelchairs
- Technique the patient is using to complete the task and any 'cheating' techniques they are using.

## Mobility

- There are a number of different ways that patients mobilise following trauma, ranging from independent walking with no aids, transfers using hoists, to slide transfers into a wheelchair.
- When first assessing a patient's mobility, it is crucial to choose the safest option.
- The choice will largely depend on a patient's age, previous mobility, injuries and doctor's instructions on weight bearing.

### Types of weight bearing

- The patient's ability to weight bear will depend on their injury and doctor's instructions.
- The physiotherapist must know how much weight the patient can take through each limb before undertaking a functional assessment.
- When determining each limb's status, plan what equipment will be needed to ensure the patient can have their mobility and function assessed.
- Examples of the types of weight bearing are outlined in Table 17.3.

### Gait patterns

- If a patient is allowed to touch weight bear or more, it is essential to assess their gait pattern during stance and swing phase.
- There will be many factors that will influence gait, such as pain, ROM, muscle tightness, splints or footdrop.
- It is important to objectively measure and document any of these factors.
- Another cause of abnormal gait after an operation could be a leg length discrepancy, which should be considered particularly following hip or pelvis surgery, but also after any type of lower limb surgery.

**Table 17.3** Main types of weight bearing encountered on a trauma unit

| Weight-bearing status | Description | Examples of Injury |
|---|---|---|
| Non-weight bearing (NWB) | No weight to be taken through the affected limb | Spiral tibial fracture Humerus fracture |
| Touch weight bearing | The patient can take only the weight of their limb through their affected limb (approximately 4–8 kg, 10–20 lb) | Acetabulum fracture Screw fixation of hip fracture |
| Partial weight bearing (PWB) | The patient can take up to 50% of their weight through their affected limb | Transverse femoral fracture |
| Full weight bearing (FWB) | The patient can take all of their weight through their affected limb | Hip replacement |

## Treatment planning

- The subjective and objective assessment findings will enable a treatment plan to be formed in consultation with the patient including the defining of SMART goals that will relate to the patient's treatment programme through to discharge from hospital and referral for outpatient physiotherapy.

## Trauma orthopaedic outpatients

- Information gathered before the assessment will assist in identifying the patient's issues, for example if the referral is from an A&E department, there may be an X-ray that can be viewed. If the referral is from an inpatient trauma team, there may be an operation note including details of the specific structures that have been operated on.

- The patient will expect the physiotherapist to know about the implications of any surgery they may have had and the prognosis relating to this, therefore it is important to become familiar with procedures and post-operative routines.

- The patient may be asked to complete outcome measure forms as they enter the department. The information provided can indicate the degree of ability/ disability that the patient feels they have as a result of their injury (Box 17.1).

### Subjective assessment

- Trauma out-patient assessment follows the standard format for out-patients (Petty 2006).

- The assessment begins at the moment the patient is first observed.

- Look at the way that they move if they have to walk in from a waiting area, the way they sit down, the way that they stand up and move in the assessment area.

- Are they using a walking aid/s? How they are using them? Are they wearing a sling or a brace?

- Gauge how much pain they are in by their body language. Non-verbal information can be as important as what the patient tells you.

- Are they following any instructions that they have been given, e.g. are they full weight bearing, when they are supposed to be touch weight bearing?

---

**Box 17.1** Examples of outcome measures

**Limbs**

Lower Extremity Function Score (LEFS) (Binkley et al 1999)

Disability of the Arm, Shoulder and Hand (DASH) (Solway et al 2002)

**Spine**

Oswestry Disability Index (ODI) (Fairbank & Pynsent 2000)

Neck Disability Index (NDI) for the cervical spine specifically (Vernon & Mior 1991)

**General**

The Patient self-efficacy score, assessment of the patient's ability to cope with their injury and pain (Bandura 1997)

---

## History of present condition

- The amount of detailed information obtained about the history of the present condition is extremely important in assisting the physiotherapist form a hypothesis, make a diagnosis and understand a patient's journey from injury to the point where they have been referred for physiotherapy out-patient management.
- The mechanism of the injury will help determine the primary diagnosis, and also how other structures may have been damaged during the accident.
- For example, the questions to ask a patient who has received a twisting injury to the knee during a game of rugby.
- How exactly did it happen?
- Which way did the knee twist?
- Was there any other force/s being applied to the leg, such as those received during a tackle from the side?
- Was there an audible noise?
- Was a 'pop', 'click' or tearing sensation felt?
- Based on this information, it may be possible to reason which structures have potentially been damaged.
- It may not be possible to gain a clear indication of the mechanism of the injuries, if for example the patient was involved in a road traffic accident, where they lost consciousness. Alternatively, they may be able to remember the accident vividly, and therefore it may distress them to talk about it in too much detail.
- It might also be helpful to establish if there are any legal proceedings following the accident. The patient may be less likely to be truthful in their answers or may display other emotions such as anger, frustration and also depression.
- If the patient is subject to a compensation claim their focus may be on the prospect of compensation rather than on their recovery.
- Each patient may have a different journey before they reach the out-patient department. The journey can indicate the extent of the issues that have been managed post injury (Figure 17.1).
- It is important to gauge what the patient has been doing between their operation or diagnosis and the start of their out-patient physiotherapy. If the patient is seen initially in a clinic setting, it may not be possible to find this out due to the time available; however, it is important that this information is obtained.
- Have they been given any exercises?
- Have they been doing them?
- How often?
- Have they been using ice or analgesia?
- Have they been following their doctor's instructions?
- If not, why not?
- The answers will indicate how compliant they have been with instructions and doing any exercises.

## Past medical history (PMH)

- The PMH may provide information about previous health issues that will help you to make decisions about how the patient may respond to treatment and any potential contraindications or precautions that need to be considered.

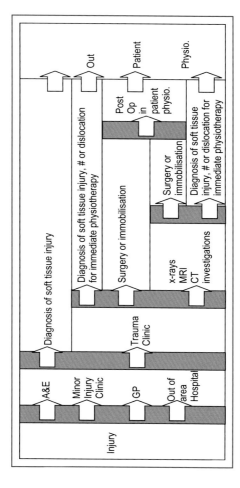

**Figure 17.1** The routes to outpatient physiotherapy.

- Table 17.4 lists some of the more common conditions that may be encountered.

## Drug history

- It is important to know what medication the patient is taking. If they are on strong analgesia such as tramadol or Oramorph, then the patient should be given a more cautious assessment, as the analgesia may be masking symptoms that may be provoked relatively easily if they were not taking pain relief.
- Note whether a patient is on anticoagulant medication, as they can bruise easily or experience bleeding into joints or soft tissue structures.
- The type of medication the patient is taking may provide a clue about the nature of their symptoms, e.g. neuroleptic medication may indicate the presence of neural pain, non-steroidal anti-inflammatory drugs (NSAIDs) may indicate that the pain is chemical in origin.
- Patients may need to be educated about how to take their medication for it to provide optimal effect, e.g. the need to take NSAIDs as an ongoing course as prescribed.

## Social history

- The social history will help to understand what the patient wants to return to and will provide information to assist the setting of treatment goals.
- When discussing the patient's work, consider if they are self-employed; how anxious they may be to get back to work. This can be difficult for the physiotherapist to manage, as often rest from work is needed after a traumatic accident, especially if is manual work. Support organisations such as the Citizen's Advice Bureau can provide practical advice to patients at this time.
- It is important to understand what a patient's job, duties and hobbies comprise so that they can be advised about when they can return to them safely. It is important to find out how regularly the patient performs any activities, particularly sports and if they have any big events coming up, such as a competition or a social event like a wedding, as this information may provide an insight into the patient's motivation.

## Body chart

- A body chart is used to chart the patient's signs and symptoms (refer to chapter 13, Figure 13.1).
- It is important to record the signs and symptoms on the first attendance, so that improvement or deterioration can be monitored. If you already have a diagnosis from the medical team then the body chart can also help you to pick out any areas of abnormal presentation that do not fit the expected clinical picture.
- Remember to tick areas that are symptom-free to get the full picture.
- The body chart can be used to record special questions, for example, with a knee injury, whether it is locking or giving way, and mark on the chart any positive or negative responses.

## Hypothesis formation

- The questioning should provide answers that assist the physiotherapist build a hypothesis about a patient's problems. The information will help determine the severity of the symptoms, the irritability and nature of the problems.

**Table 17.4** Examples of conditions and factors to be considered when planning an assessment

| Condition | Potential effect on patient's management and adaptations to treatment |
|---|---|
| Hypothyroid | Can easily fatigue, if not controlled. e.g. may benefit from having a Zimmer frame as well as elbow crutches at home, if non-weight bearing |
| Heart and chest problems | Over exertion may cause problems such as shortness of breath or angina, e.g. reduce duration and difficulty of treatment to avoid this and ensure that they replicate this at home |
| Rheumatoid arthritis | May have pains in multiple joints, e.g. may need Fischer crutches for mobility. Avoid excessive loading of joints to avoid exacerbation |
| Diabetes | Can cause slow healing of bone, soft tissues and wounds. Ensure wounds are being monitored carefully by GP (or by a health care professional trained to deal with wound care). Treatment progression can be delayed as a result |
| Use of long-term steroids | Can cause thinning to the skin and ligaments to become weaker. Be careful with soft tissue work, such as cross friction massage |
| Previous injury to same area – must also ask if the patient had physiotherapy treatment after this injury. This can indicate how well patient may respond to repeating certain treatment modalities | Fractures – outcome may be worse as the joint and soft tissues will have old scar tissue and damage, causing increased stiffness<br>Sprains – need to make sure that proprioception training is included in treatment to try to stop recurrent problems<br>Dislocations – recurrent dislocations usually need surgery, therefore this needs to be discussed with the surgical/medical team or GP |
| Previous injury to different area | Previous fractures to opposite leg or to upper limbs can affect a patient's ability to use walking aids. This also applies to patients with osteoarthritis<br>A number of previous fractures may suggest that the patient needs to be tested for osteoporosis |

## Objective assessment

- The objective assessment should be used to confirm or disprove the hypothesis and should be planned with this in mind.
- Having completed the subjective assessment, the patient will need to be appropriately undressed to enable affected areas to be seen clearly.

### Observation

- Observe the patient's posture, the way that they are moving and the way they are holding the injured body part. Consider the patient generally before looking more closely at specific areas.
- Is the patient wearing a brace, sling or Tubigrip correctly.
- Look at the soft tissues.
- Is the area swollen?
- If so where?
- Is there bruising or redness?
- If so where?
- If the skin is red, is it associated with a wound?
- If a wound is present, is it dressed and can this be removed?
- Are stitches still in situ? (consider if the redness and swelling is due to inflammation or infection).
- When noticing these things, it is important to think about why they are there. Does it tie in with the method of injury, diagnosis or with the surgery that they have had? If it does, then it may limit the amount of assessment the patient can tolerate.
- Is there any noticeable deformity. If it is an acute injury, then a brief assessment may be warranted before the patient is referred for further investigations, such as an X-ray or scan.
- Deformity may be present post medical intervention, but has been examined and is determined not to be detrimental to their function. This is often the case with a distal radius fracture in the elderly, where they are managed conservatively in a cast and have a deformity after the fracture is healed. The patient usually returns to full pain-free function despite this.

### Palpation

- Patients can often be nervous of having their injured limb handled, due to pain and anxiety that the injury may be made worse. It is important to warn a patient prior to palpating their affected body part and obtain their consent; it is part of the process of the patient learning to trust their therapist.
- Start the palpation by using the back of the hand to feel the affected area. This allows perception of any increased temperature and swelling in a way that looks less provocative from the patient's perspective. It will indicate how much pain the patient gets on light palpation, which will guide further handling during the assessment.
- Patients can be given a VAS scale to show how much pain they feel during palpation (Wewers & Lowe 1990). If they are in no or minimal pain, then firmer palpation may be tolerated, to enable identification of the injured tissues, swelling, and any deformity that is not evident on observation alone.

TRAUMA ORTHOPAEDICS

17

275

## Precautions

- Having observed and palpated the area, ensure that there are no obvious limitations to the patient's ROM, or specific instructions from a surgeon, e.g. following a proximal fracture of the humerus a patient has been told they can lift their arm to shoulder height (90° flexion and abduction). The physiotherapist should not consider assessing the full range into elevation, due to the stress this will place on the fracture site.

- In the cases where the patient is strictly non-weight bearing, it may be inappropriate to assess the patient's muscle strength, as this may overload the joint or fracture.

- Assessment planning should take into account these types of issues. This may mean that the planned assessment may be limited, e.g. to assess ROM, respecting the patient's pain, following postoperative instructions or respecting inflammation around the joint.

- It is better to assess less and maintain the patient's confidence, than to assess too much and cause the patient unnecessary pain, which could detrimentally affect the therapist–patient relationship. There should always be the opportunity to get the patient back in, to continue the assessment.

- It may be necessary to give the patient instructions about rest, ice, NSAIDs and get them to return when inflammation has been reduced.

## Range of movement

- The following information should be noted during the assessment of active and passive joint movement:
- The quality of the movement
- The range of movement
- The presence of resistance through the range of movement and at the end of the range of movement
- Pain behaviour (local and referred) through the range
- The occurrence of muscle spasm during the range of movement (Petty 2006).

- This information should confirm that structures are damaged, or whether they are tight or lengthened, weak or overactive. This will help you to build a clinical picture of what is causing the patient's symptoms. The use of passive ROM and gentle overpressure (if end range is achievable) can be used if the patient's symptoms are not severe and irritable, to assess the integrity of the soft tissues, especially ligaments (Hengeveld and Banks 2005).

## Muscle testing

- After any injury the muscles are likely to become weak or tight, usually due to immobilisation in casts or braces or due to pain. It is important to note the strength in inner, middle and outer range, to determine specific functional weakness and to enable treatment to target the specific needs of the muscles.

- Muscle length is often affected post injury, and can cause biomechanical problems, leading to prolonged pain and decreased function.

## Neurological testing

- Diagnostic neurological testing will be required if the patient has nerve injuries caused by specific fractures, burns or lacerating trauma.

- After prolonged immobilisation the mobility of the nervous system can become reduced in the injured area, which can cause neurogenic symptoms. Testing neurodynamics will provide diagnostic information about the problems being encountered by the neural tissue (Petty 2006).

- If a patient presents with neurological symptoms it is important to know why this is happening. A patient may be getting paraesthesia (pins and needles) if their cast is too tight, which will need to be referred to the plaster room as soon as possible.

- Alternatively they may have skin numbness around their wound, where a superficial cutaneous nerve has been cut during surgery.

- It is also important to bear in mind that paraesthesia distal to a very swollen and inflamed joint, may be due to the nerves being compressed. It is essential that nerve compression is reduced as soon as possible.

- In the case of compartment syndrome, rapid surgery is required to release tight fascial compartments. Conditions such as deep vein thrombosis (DVT) will also need immediate medical attention.

- Nerve palsies are common with injuries such as humeral shaft fractures, and Achilles tendon ruptures. The presentation will vary from patient to patient, so a detailed neurological assessment will be required to map the extent of the injury.

- Refer to the assessment of nerve damage in Chapter 4.

## Joint integrity tests and special tests

- There are a number or joint integrity and special tests for each joint, e.g. Lachman's test for anterior cruciate ligament instability. These tests are useful for diagnosing soft tissue injuries.

- With an acute injury it can be difficult, if not impossible, to perform some of these tests due to the patient's pain, swelling or muscle spasm.

- Manage the acute signs and symptoms and bring the patient back to continue the assessment once pain and swelling have reduced.

## Accessory testing

- Accessory movements can be used to assess the articular structures, generally after the acute phase. They can assess hypomobility or hypermobility, and pain presenting throughout the range of joint motion (Maitland et al, 2005).

## Gait

- Patients need to be able to mobilise safely at all stages of their treatment and will require guidance about how to progress to walking unaided with a reciprocal gait pattern.

- Some considerations that need to be noted during gait assessment are listed in Table 17.5.

## Psychological assessment

- In the assessment and treatment of trauma patients there may be the presentation of emotions such as anger, frustration and depression at any stage in their management.

- It is important to listen to the patient, and involve specialists in the management of psychological issues for advice.

- Refer to Chapter 16 for additional information on the management of the psychological effects of trauma.

**Table 17.5** Gait pattern, observations and considerations

| Gait pattern | Observation and questions |
|---|---|
| Non-weight bearing with frame or crutches | Are they coping with their walking aid – are they safe? Posture – is their trunk flexed – are their crutches/frame the right height? Are they hopping through too far? Do they need to non-weight bear? Are they in too much pain or too afraid to weight bear? |
| Partial weight bearing – 50% with frame or crutches | Are they putting the right amount of weight through their limb? This can be checked by weighing the patient and then checking them weight bearing through the scales Are they using heel–toe gait pattern? If not, why not? Can you correct this? Are they supposed to be using a boot? Or would they benefit from more support from a brace to their knee or ankle? |
| Full weight bearing with crutches | See above |
| Full weight bearing without aids | Do they have an antalgic gait? Do they need to be using a crutch on the contralateral side or two crutches to improve this? Do they have a Trendelenburg gait? Do they have a leg length discrepancy or a drop foot? |

## Treatment planning

- Following the assessment, the treatment plan can be agreed with the patient and appropriate treatment goals and targets can be established.
- Problem-orientated medical records or SOAP formats are commonly used for identifying goals and indicators that can be used to monitor progress.

The references for this chapter can be found on www.expertconsult.com.

Page numbers followed by "f" indicate figures, "t" indicate tables, and "b" indicate boxes.

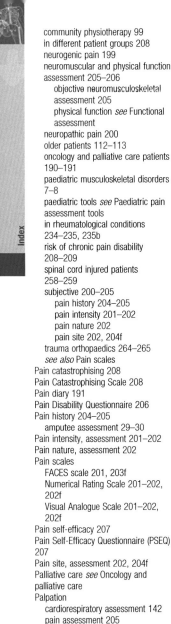

Printed in the United States
By Bookmasters